An Imaging Atlas of
Human Anatomy

J. Weir
MB, BS, DMRD, FRCP(Ed), FRCR
Professor of Radiology
Department of Diagnostic Radiology
University of Aberdeen

P.H. Abrahams
MB, BS
Senior Lecturer in Clinical Anatomy
Department of Anatomy and Developmental Biology
University College
London

with six contributors

A-M. Belli
MB, BS, DMRD, FRCR
Senior Lecturer and Honorary Consultant Radiologist
Royal Postgraduate Medical School
Hammersmith Hospital
London

A.P. Hemingway
BSc, MB, BS, DMRD, FRCR, FRCP
Professor of Diagnostic Radiology
Academic Department of Radiology
University of Sheffield

M.D. Hourihan
MB, BCh, FRCR
Consultant Neuroradiologist
Department of Radiology
University Hospital of Wales

N.R. Moore
MA, MB, BChir, MRCP, FRCR
Lecturer in Radiology
Department of Radiology
University of Oxford

G. Needham
BSc, MB, ChB, FRCR
Consultant Radiologist
Aberdeen Royal Infirmary
Aberdeen

J.P. Owen
MB, BS, DMRD, FRCR
Senior Lecturer and Honorary Consultant Radiologist
Department of Radiology
University of Newcastle upon Tyne

Wolfe Publishing Ltd

Copyright © 1992 Wolfe Publishing Ltd.
Published by Wolfe Publishing Ltd, 1992
Printed by BPCC Hazells Ltd, Aylesbury, England
ISBN 0 7234 1669 9 (Hard cover)
ISBN 0 7234 1694 X (Soft cover)
Reprinted 1992

A CIP catalogue record for this book is available from the British
Library.

For a full list of forthcoming titles and details of our surgical, dental and
veterinary atlases, please write to Mosby–Year Book Europe Ltd,
Brook House, 2–16 Torrington Place, London WC1E 7LT, England.

Contents

Acknowledgements

Professor D.J. Allison, Hammersmith Hospital, London (Fig. B, p.132 and Fig. B, p.135).

Dr A. Clifton, Atkinson Morley's Hospital, London (Fig. B, p.68).

Dr D.C. Cumberland, Sheffield (Figs A–F, p.103).

Dr J. Jackson, Hammersmith Hospital, London (Fig. A, p.135).

Dr I.W. McCall, Robert Jones and Agnes Hunt Hospital, Oswestry (Fig. A, p.68).

Dr S.A. Russell, St Mary's Hospital, Manchester (Figs A–D, p.49 and Figs A–D, p.50).

Miss Elaine Sassoon (FRCS), UCL Department of Plastic Surgery, London (Fig. B, p.30).

Preface

Imaging methods used to display normal human anatomy have improved dramatically over the last few decades. The ability to demonstrate the soft tissues by using the modern technologies of magnetic resonance imaging, X-ray computed tomography, and ultrasound has greatly facilitated our understanding of the link between anatomy as shown in the dissecting room and that necessary for clinical practice. This Atlas has been produced because of the new technology and the fundamental changes that are occurring in the teaching of anatomy. It enables the preclinical medical student to relate to basic anatomy while, at the same time, providing a comprehensive study guide for the clinical interpretation of imaging, applicable for all undergraduate and postgraduate levels.

Several distinguished authors, experts in their own fields of imaging, have contributed to this book, which has benefited from editorial integration to ensure balance and cohesion. The Atlas is designed to complement and supplement the *Colour Atlas of Human Anatomy* by McMinn (Wolfe Publishing Ltd).

Duplication of images occurs only where it is necessary to demonstrate anatomical points of interest or difficulty. Similarly, examples of different imaging modalities of the same anatomical region are only included if they contribute to a better understanding of the region shown. Radiographs that show important landmarks in limb ossification centre development, together with examples of some common congenital anomalies, are also documented. In certain sections, notably MR and CT, the legends may cover more than one page, so that a specific structure can be followed in continuity through various levels and planes.

Human anatomy does not alter, but our methods of demonstrating it have changed significantly. Modern imaging allows certain structures and their relationships to be seen for the first time, and this has aided us in their interpretation. Knowledge and understanding of radiological anatomy are fundamental to all those involved in patient care, from the nurse and the paramedic to medical students and clinicians.

Dedication

To all our families and, particularly, to the
children conceived and born during the production
of this Atlas

Introduction

Angiography

Access to the arterial system in order to produce an arteriogram (angiogram) is usually obtained by puncture and catheterisation of a femoral artery under local anaesthesia. Radiographic contrast medium is then injected into the vessel in the area under examination. If, for some reason, access via the femoral artery is not possible (e.g., owing to iliac occlusive disease or the presence of a graft), alternative sites, such as the brachial or axillary artery, can be used. Translumbar aortography (TLA), a method of arteriography that involves direct percutaneous puncture of the aorta, is now less commonly employed as it does not allow selective catheterisation of aortic branches and hence percutaneous interventional vascular procedures cannot be performed. The development of new technology has meant that the aorta and the main upper and lower limb arteries can be visualised from an intravenous injection of contrast medium (into the brachial vein, superior vena cava, or right atrium), obviating the need for arterial puncture in some patients. This technique employs digital subtraction angiography (DSA), whereby unwanted background information is 'subtracted', leaving only an image of the blood vessels. Images of arteries obtained by injection into a vein are referred to as intravenous DSA examinations (IV DSA). DSA images of arteries can, of course, be obtained by direct intra-arterial injection (IA DSA).

Manual photographic subtraction of background information can also be performed with conventional (nondigital) arteriography. Subtraction, either photographic or digital, is used in cases in which fine vascular detail is required and can be simply recognised by the fact that, in contrast to an unsubtracted film, the arteries appear black as opposed to white. Different radiographic projections are sometimes employed to visualise best the vasculature, e.g., in the aortic arch an anteroposterior view may not clearly show the origins of the vessels arising from the arch as they are very close to each other and may be superimposed. A left anterior oblique position opens the arch, allowing better visualisation of the origins of the brachiocephalic, left carotid and subclavian arteries. The angiograms in this book use the anteroposterior (AP) projection, unless otherwise indicated.

The veins may be visualised in the same way as the arteries, e.g., by direct puncture and catheterisation (via the femoral vein in most instances). The veins of the upper and lower limbs are imaged by injecting contrast medium via an 18G or 20G needle placed in a peripheral vein, e.g. the dorsum of the foot or hand, or the antecubital fossa. Alternatively, if imaging from an arterial injection over a prolonged period of time, the arterial, capillary and venous phases can be recorded and venous anatomy visualised. This is a particularly useful way of imaging the portal venous system without necessitating direct trans-splenic or transhepatic puncture.

For arterial puncture, catheterisation and imaging techniques, and for details of the type of equipment used in angiography, specialised texts should be consulted.

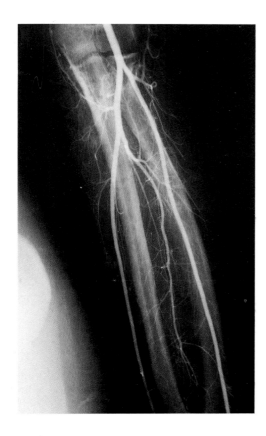

Brachial arteriogram demonstrating the forearm arteries. There is no subtraction, as shown by the presence of the forearm bones in the radiograph.

Computed Tomography

The limitation of all plain radiographic techniques is the two-dimensional representation of a three-dimensional structure. The linear attenuation coefficients of all of the tissues in the X-ray beam form the image.

Computed tomography (CT) obtains a series of different angular X-ray projections which are processed by a computer to give a section of specified thickness. The CT image comprises a regular matrix of picture elements (pixels). All of the tissues contained within the pixel attenuate the X-ray projections and result in a mean attenuation value for the pixel. This value is compared with the attenuation value of water and is displayed on a scale (the Hounsfield scale). Water is defined as 0 Hounsfield units (HU) and the scale is 2,000 HU wide. Air typically has a HU number of −1,000; fat is approximately −100 HU; soft tissues are in the range +20 to +70 HU, and bone is greater than +400 HU.

The CT machine consists of a rigid metal frame with an X-ray tube sited opposite a set of detectors. In early designs the tube and detectors scanned across the patient and then rotated to a different position ('translate–rotate'). Current third-generation CT machines have a wider detector array and an X-ray fan beam, which encompasses the whole patient. All the views per slice can be collected simultaneously so that the tube and detectors only rotate around the patient. Routine acquisition times are 2–4 seconds, although a variant of the design utilises a constantly rotating tube/detector system which permits subsecond scan times.

All CT machines, of whatever generation, share similar components. The detectors are either gas ionisation chambers, or scintillation crystals linked to photomultiplier tubes. The signal is digitised by an analogue to digital converter (ADC) in the gantry. The digitised signal is transferred to the image processing computer and subsequently displayed on the operator's console. Images are usually photographed on medical recording film (hard copy) using optical or laser cameras. For long-term storage, the data is transferred to magnetic media (tape or disc) or to optical disc.

No specific preparation is required for examinations of the brain, spine, musculoskeletal system and chest. Studies of the abdomen and pelvis almost always require opacification of the gastrointestinal tract, using a solution of dilute contrast medium (either water-soluble or a barium compound). Generally, 750–1,000 ml are given orally 30–60 minutes prior to imaging, with the final 300 ml taken as the patient enters the examination room. The large bowel may also be opacified by a solution of contrast medium administered rectally, either in a preparation room or on the CT table. Examinations of the female pelvis are often performed after the insertion of a vaginal tampon to facilitate interpretation.

Identification of vascular structures may be made on the basis of anatomy alone, but the intravenous injection of water-soluble contrast medium may be required. Techniques vary according to the individual case, but the most common method is to inject a bolus of 50 ml followed by a rapid infusion of 50 ml, using contrast medium of 300–370 mg iodine/ml.

Generally, all studies are performed with the patient supine, and images are obtained in the transverse plane. Modern CT machines allow up to 25° of gantry angulation, which is particularly valuable in spinal imaging. Occasionally, coronal images are obtained in the investigation of cranial abnormalities; in these cases the patient lies prone, with the neck extended, and the gantry is angled appropriately.

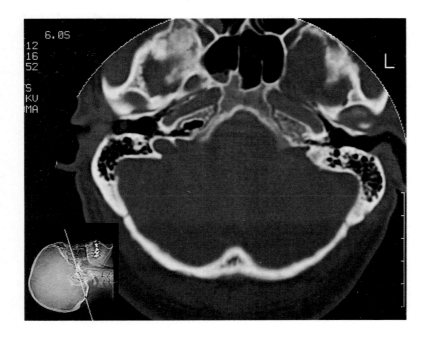

Axial CT scan through the base of the skull, at the level of the external auditory meati. Bone window settings have been used to demonstrate the skull base.

Magnetic Resonance Imaging

Magnetic resonance imaging (MRI) combines a strong magnetic field and radiofrequency (RF) energy to study the distribution and behaviour of hydrogen protons in fat and water.

The spinning proton of the hydrogen nucleus can be thought of as a tiny bar magnet, with a north and south pole. In the absence of an external magnetic field, the magnetic moments of all of the protons in the body are randomly arranged. However, when the patient is placed in a strong magnetic field these magnetic moments align either with or against the field lines of the magnet. There is a small excess of magnetic moments which align with the field so that a net magnetic vector is established.

RF energy is used to generate a second magnetic field, perpendicular to the static magnetic field of the machine. The result of this second magnetic field is to rotate or 'flip' the protons away from the static magnetic field; the amount of rotation depends on the quantity of RF energy absorbed. Once the RF field is switched off, the protons experience only the effects of the static magnetic field and flip back to their original position. During this return to equilibrium, a process which is called 'relaxation', protons emit the RF energy which they had acquired. This energy is detected by the antenna in the MRI machine, digitised, amplified, and, finally, spatially encoded by the array processor. The resulting images are displayed on the operator's console and can be recorded on hard copy (for viewing) or transferred to magnetic tape or optical disc (for storage).

MRI systems are graded according to the strength of the magnetic field they produce. High-field systems are those capable of producing a magnetic field strength of 1–2 Tesla (T) (10,000–20,000 Gauss), mid-field systems operate at 0.35–0.5 T, and low-field systems produce a field strength of less than 0.2 T. Mid- and high-field systems use superconducting magnets in which the coils of copper wire are kept in a superconducting state ($-269°C$) by being immersed in an insulated helium bath. Electromagnets are fitted in resistive systems and are limited by heating factors to 0.35 T. The third type uses permanently magnetised metal cores and is of low field strength.

MRI does not cause any recognised biological hazard. Patients who have any form of pacemaker or implanted electro-inductive device must not be examined. Other prohibited items include ferromagnetic intracranial aneurysm clips, certain types of cardiac valve replacement, and intra-ocular metallic foreign bodies. Generally, it is safe to examine patients who have extracranial vascular clips and orthopaedic prostheses, but these may cause local artefacts. Loose metal items must be excluded from the examination room.

The preparation for an MRI examination is simple. Patients wear metal-free clothes and must answer a rigorous safety questionnaire. Antiperistaltic agents (e.g., parenteral hyoscine N-butylbromide or glucagon) are often used in abdominal and pelvic examinations. Software techniques counteract respiratory motion for chest and abdominal imaging. Electrocardiogram (ECG) gating is used for cardiac studies.

MR images may be obtained in any orthogonal or non-orthogonal plane. There is a wide range of pulse sequences, each of which provides a different image contrast. An intravenous injection of contrast medium (a gadolinium complex) may be given to enhance tumours, and inflammatory and vascular abnormalities.

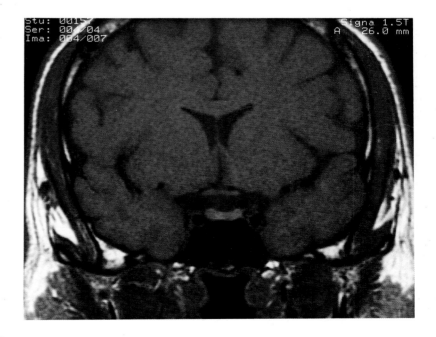

Coronal MR image of the brain, through the lateral ventricles.

Ultrasound

In contrast with the other images in this book, ultrasound images do not depend on the use of electromagnetic wave forms. It is the properties of high-frequency sound waves (longitudinal waves) and their interaction with biological tissues that go to form these 'echograms'.

A sound wave of appropriate frequency (diagnostic range 3.5–10 MHz) is produced by piezo-electric principles. Both the size and shape of the emitting crystal and its resonant frequency are important factors in determining the course of the sound beam within the tissues to be examined.

As the beam passes through tissues, two important effects determine image production. These are attenuation and reflection. Attenuation is caused by the loss of energy from the system, due to absorption and reflection, refraction and beam divergence out of the range of the receiver. The greater the attenuation of the sound beam through the tissue, the lower the resultant signal intensity received. Reflection of sound waves within the range of the receiver produces the image, the texture of which is dependent upon differences in acoustic impedance between different tissues. Ultrasound imaging systems are sensitive to the very small changes in acoustic impedance within soft tissue.

Through the application of these basic principles, sophisticated hardware has been developed that converts the pulse–echo system, briefly described above, into a real-time two-dimensional sectional image. The addition of the facility to measure blood-flow direction and velocity ultrasonically (using the Doppler principle) has led to the development and wide availability of duplex scanners.

The effects of shadowing and enhancement within an ultrasound image are of paramount importance. Systems are designed assuming an average attenuation through a depth of tissue, and are balanced to give an even intensity of signal for deep and superficial tissues. An acoustic shadow occurs when a tissue within the measured depth has a higher than average attenuation; all tissues deep to this will appear with a falsely lower intensity (shadowed). Conversely, a tissue with a lower than average attenuation will cause all tissues deep to this to appear falsely high in intensity (enhanced). Fibrous tissue, calcification and gas all produce acoustic shadows, whereas fluid-filled structures often cause enhancement.

If a selection of ultrasound transducers with varying frequencies, focusing mechanisms, and shapes and sizes is available, visualisation of a wide range of tissues, from the neonatal brain to the soft tissues of the hand, becomes possible. Only relevant ultrasound images have been included in the book to illustrate a particular point or area, as the real-time nature of ultrasound precludes further coverage. Interpretation of the anatomy by static ultrasound images is more difficult than that by other imaging modalities because the technique is highly operator dependent and provides different information on tissue structure and form than other imaging methods.

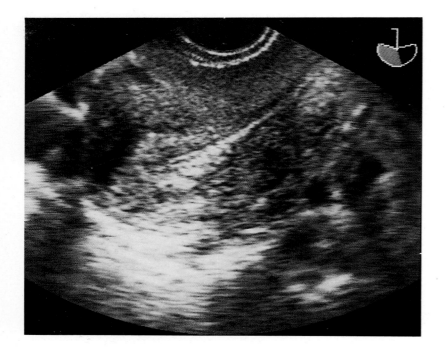

Transvaginal ultrasound scan of the uterus, in a longitudinal plane. The high frequency (7.5 MHz) probe is placed in the upper vagina in order to obtain this tissue detail.

Head, neck and brain

A Skull. Occipitofrontal projection

1 Frontal sinus
2 Sagittal suture
3 Crista galli
4 Lambdoid suture
5 Petrous part of temporal bone
6 Internal acoustic meatus
7 Mastoid process
8 Basi-occiput
9 Lateral mass of atlas (first cervical vertebra)
10 Odontoid process (dens) of axis (second cervical vertebra)
11 Floor of maxillary sinus (antrum)
12 Nasal septum
13 Sella turcica
14 Ethmoidal air cells
15 Superior orbital fissure
16 Temporal surface of greater wing ⎫
17 Body   ⎬ of sphenoid
18 Lesser wing   ⎭
19 Foramen rotundum

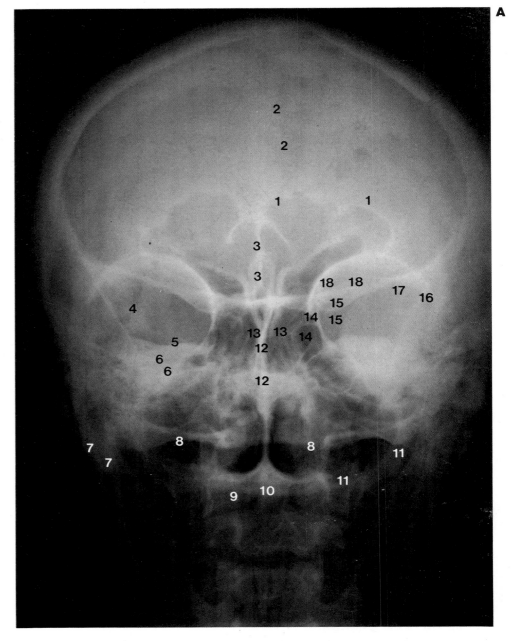

**B Skull, demonstrating the foramina rotunda.
Occipitofrontal projection**

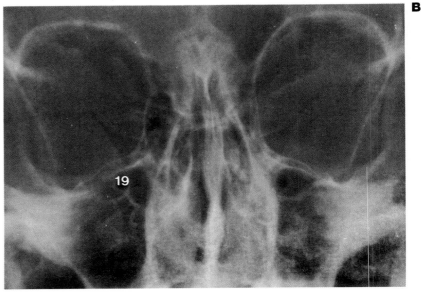

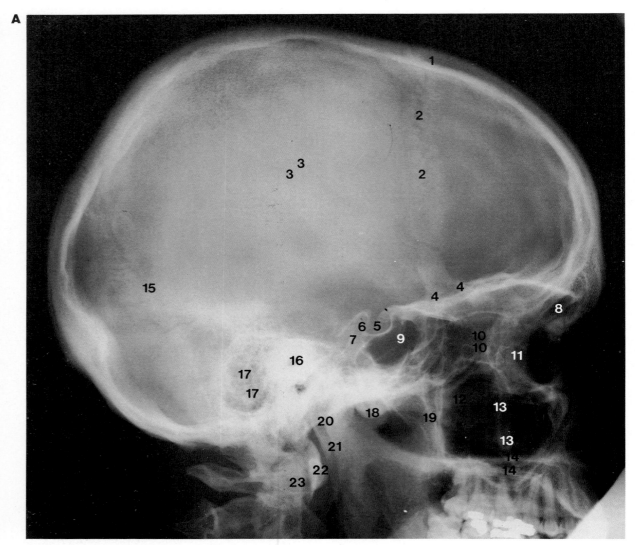

1	Diploë
2	Coronal suture
3	Grooves for middle meningeal vessels
4	Greater wing of sphenoid
5	Pituitary fossa (sella turcica)
6	Dorsum sellae
7	Clivus
8	Frontal sinus
9	Sphenoidal sinus
10	Ethmoidal air cells
11	Frontal process } of zygoma
12	Arch
13	Maxillary process } of maxilla
14	Palatine process
15	Lambdoid suture
16	External acoustic meatus
17	Mastoid air cells
18	Articular tubercle for temporomandibular joint
19	Coronoid process } of mandible
20	Condyle
21	Ramus
22	Anterior arch of atlas (first cervical vertebra)
23	Odontoid process (dens) of axis (second cervical vertebra)
24	Posterior } clinoid process
25	Anterior
26	Tuberculum sellae
27	Planum sphenoidale
28	Carotid sulcus
29	Basilar part of occipital bone
30	Middle clinoid process

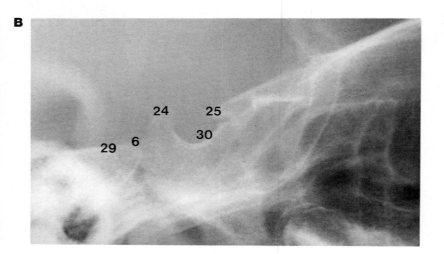

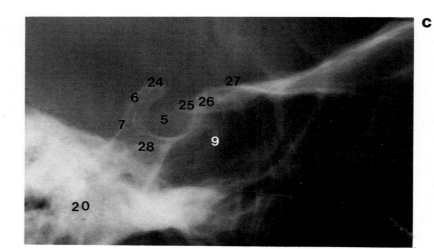

Pituitary fossa (sella turcica), **B** of a 7-year-old child, **C** of a 23-year-old woman. Lateral projections

Skull. 30° fronto-occipital (Townes') projection

1 Sagittal suture
2 Coronal suture
3 Lambdoid suture
4 Foramen magnum
5 Dorsum sellae
6 Odontoid process (dens) of axis (second cervical vertebra)
7 Arch of atlas (first cervical vertebra)
8 Zygomatic arch
9 Mandibular condyle
10 Internal acoustic meatus
11 Superior semicircular canal
12 Arcuate eminence ⎫ of temporal
13 Petrous part ⎭ bone

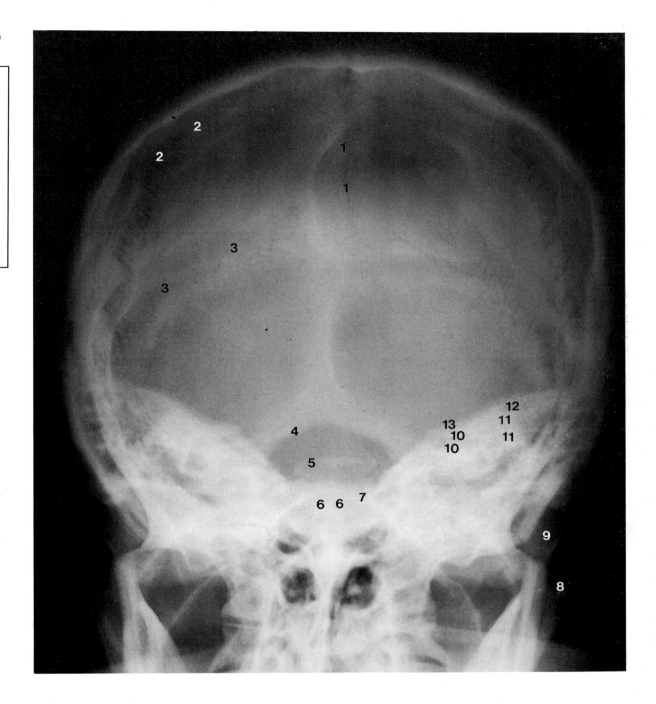

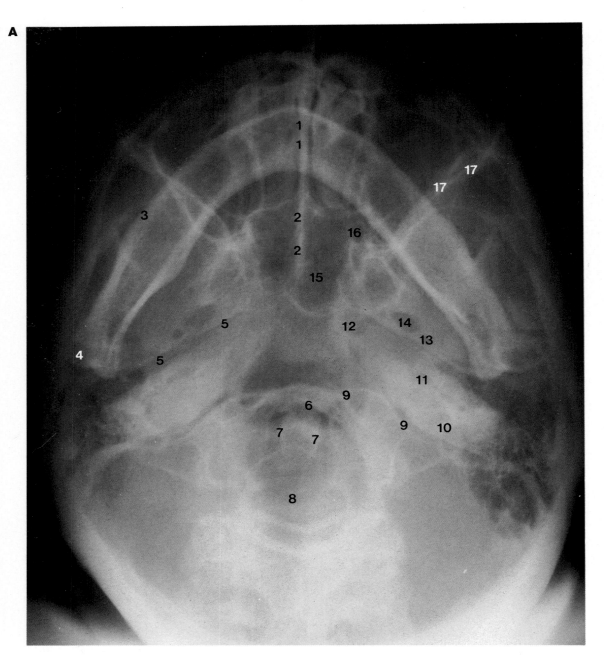

A Skull. Submentovertical projection

1	Perpendicular plate of ethmoid
2	Vomer
3	Body ⎫ of mandible
4	Head ⎭
5	Auditory (Eustachian) tube
6	Anterior arch of atlas (first cervical vertebra)
7	Odontoid process (dens) of axis (second cervical vertebra)
8	Foramen magnum
9	Occipital condyle
10	Jugular foramen
11	Carotid canal
12	Foramen lacerum
13	Foramen spinosum
14	Foramen ovale
15	Sphenoidal sinus
16	Greater palatine foramen
17	Greater wing of sphenoid (forming posterior orbital margin)
18	Zygomatic bone
19	Temporal process of zygomatic bone
20	Zygomatic process of temporal bone

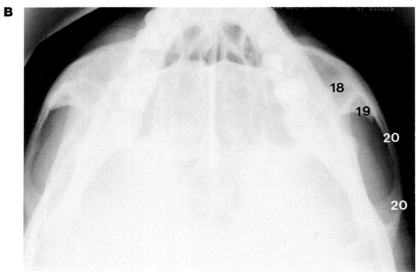

B Skull, with additional angulation for zygomatic arches. Submentovertical projection

A

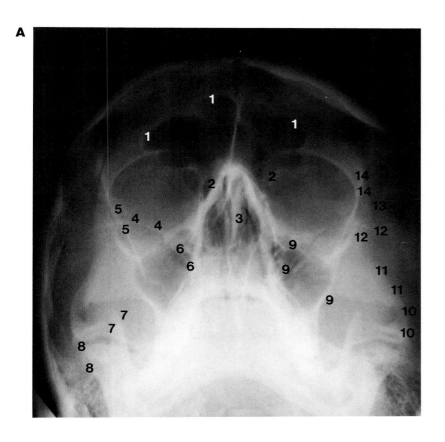

B

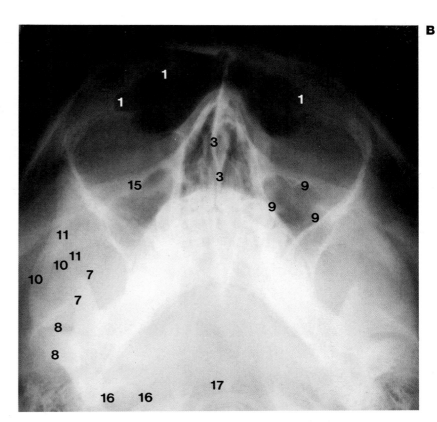

Facial bones and paranasal sinuses, A occipitofrontal projection, **B** occipitomental projection, **C** lateral projection

1	Frontal sinuses
2	Ethmoidal sinuses
3	Nasal septum
4	Lesser ⎫
5	Greater ⎬ wing of sphenoid
6	Superior orbital fissure
7	Coronoid process ⎫
8	Condyle ⎬ of mandible
9	Left maxillary sinus (antrum)
10	Zygomatic process of temporal bone
11	Temporal ⎫
12	Frontal ⎬ process of zygomatic bone
13	Frontozygomatic suture
14	Zygomatic process of frontal bone
15	Infra-orbital foramen
16	Right jugular foramen
17	Anterior arch of atlas (first cervical vertebra)
18	Sphenoidal sinus
19	Sella turcica
20	Posterior ⎫
21	Anterior ⎬ wall of maxillary sinus (antrum)
22	Horizontal plate of palatine bone
23	Palatine ⎫
24	Malar ⎬ process of maxilla

C

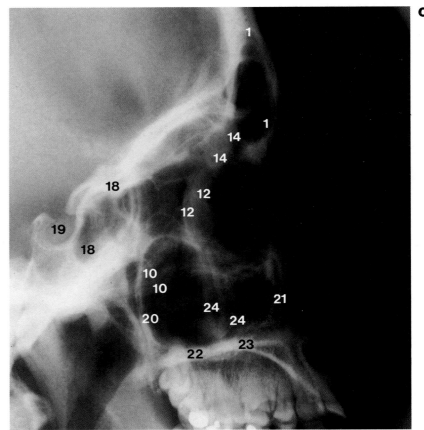

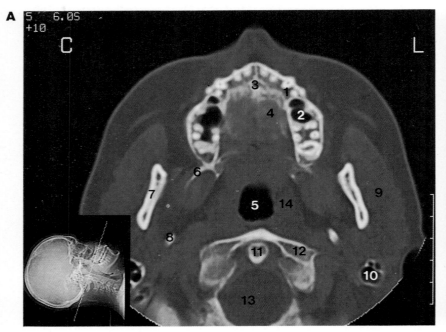

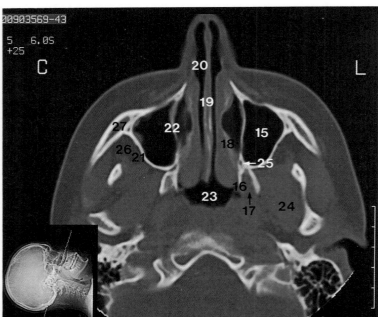

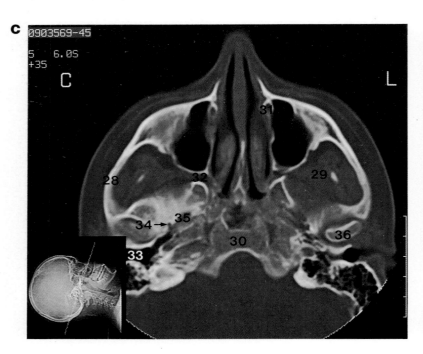

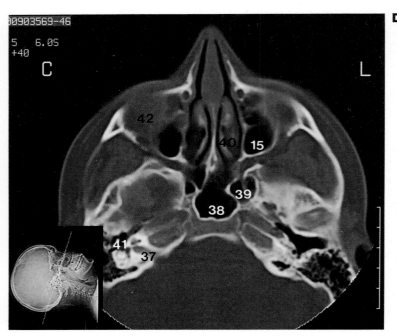

Facial bones and paranasal sinuses. Axial CT images are demonstrated at the following levels: **A** hard palate; **B** inferior nasal turbinate; **C** maxillary sinus; **D** middle turbinates; **E** ethmoidal sinuses; **F** ethmoidal sinuses and upper sphenoidal sinus; **G** optic nerve; **H** frontal sinus

1	Alveolar rim	11	Odontoid process (dens)	21	Lateral wall ⎫ of maxillary sinus (antrum)
2	Alveolar recess	12	Anterior arch of atlas (first cervical vertebra)	22	Medial wall ⎭
3	Incisive canal	13	Spinal canal	23	Nasopharynx
4	Hard palate	14	Deglutitional muscles	24	Lateral pterygoid muscle
5	Oropharynx	15	Maxillary sinus (antrum)	25	Greater palatine canal
6	Lateral pterygoid plate	16	Medial pterygoid plate	26	Infratemporal fossa
7	Ramus of mandible	17	Pterygoid fossa	27	Zygoma
8	Styloid process	18	Inferior nasal concha (turbinate)	28	Zygomatic arch
9	Masseter muscle	19	Vomer	29	Temporalis muscle
10	Mastoid process	20	Nasal cavity	30	Clivus (basi-occipital bone)

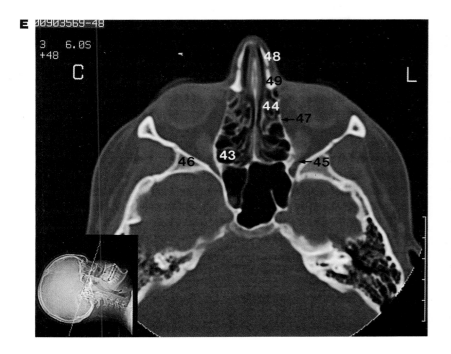

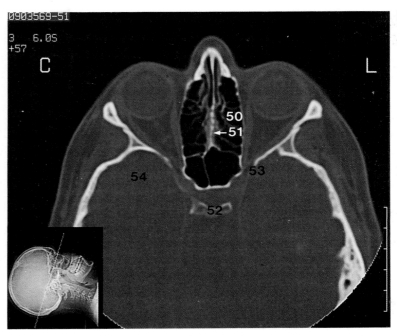

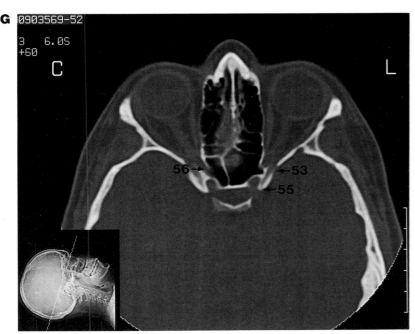

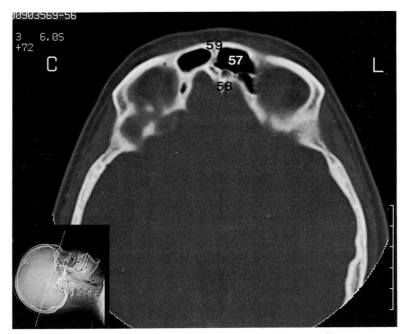

31	Nasolacrimal duct	41	Middle ear cavity	51	Perpendicular plate of ethmoid bone
32	Pterygopalatine fossa	42	Globe	52	Dorsum sellae
33	External acoustic canal	43	Posterior } ethmoidal air cells	53	Superior orbital fissure
34	Foramen spinosum	44	Anterior }	54	Temporal lobe
35	Foramen ovale	45	Inferior orbital fissure	55	Anterior clinoid process
36	Mandibular condyle	46	Greater wing of sphenoid	56	Optic canal
37	Internal acoustic meatus	47	Lamina papyracea	57	Frontal sinus
38	Sphenoidal sinus	48	Nasal bone	58	Crista galli
39	Inferolateral recess	49	Lacrimal bone	59	Frontal bone
40	Middle concha (turbinate)	50	Middle ethmoidal air cells		

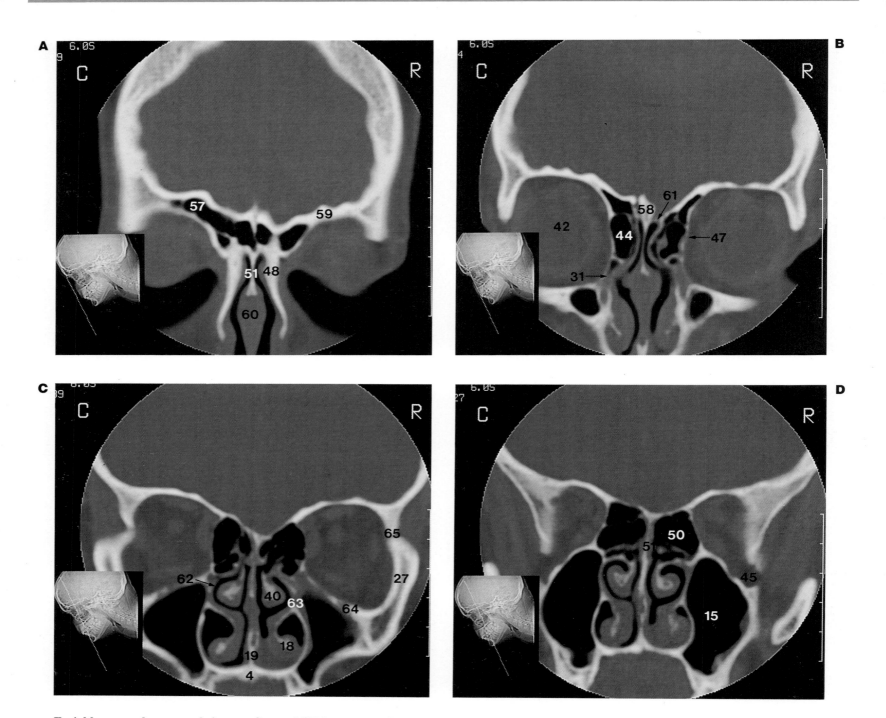

Facial bones and paranasal sinuses. Coronal CT images are demonstrated at the following levels: **A** frontal sinus; **B** anterior maxillary sinus and ethmoidal sinuses; **C** middle ethmoidal sinus and maxillary sinus; **D** middle maxillary sinus; **E** posterior ethmoidal sinus; **F** posterior maxillary sinus; **G** anterior sphenoidal sinus; **H** posterior sphenoidal sinus

1	Alveolar rim	13	Spinal canal	25	Greater palatine canal
2	Alveolar recess	14	Deglutitional muscles	26	Infratemporal fossa
3	Incisive canal	15	Maxillary sinus (antrum)	27	Zygoma
4	Hard palate	16	Medial pterygoid plate	28	Zygomatic arch
5	Oropharynx	17	Pterygoid fossa	29	Temporalis muscle
6	Lateral pterygoid plate	18	Inferior nasal concha (turbinate)	30	Clivus (basi-occipital bone)
7	Ramus of mandible	19	Vomer	31	Nasolacrimal duct
8	Styloid process	20	Nasal cavity	32	Pterygopalatine fossa
9	Masseter muscle	21	Lateral wall ⎫ of maxillary sinus (antrum)	33	External acoustic canal
10	Mastoid process	22	Medial wall ⎭	34	Foramen spinosum
11	Odontoid process (dens)	23	Nasopharynx	35	Foramen ovale
12	Anterior arch of atlas (first cervical vertebra)	24	Lateral pterygoid muscle	36	Mandibular condyle

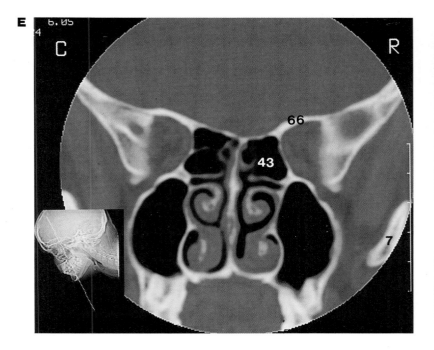

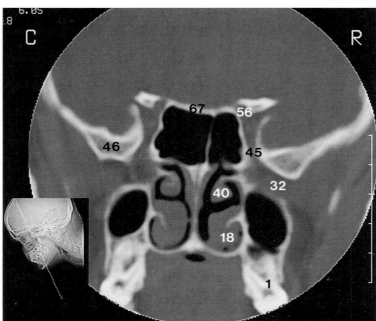

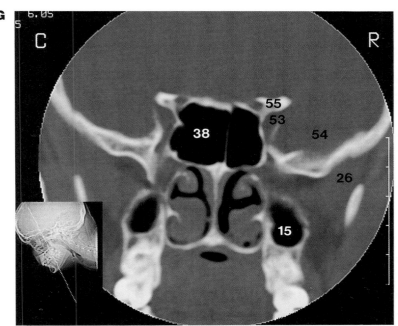

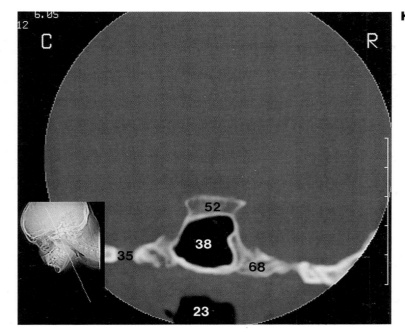

37	Internal acoustic meatus	48	Nasal bone	59	Frontal bone
38	Sphenoidal sinus	49	Lacrimal bone	60	Cartilaginous portion of nasal septum
39	Inferolateral recess	50	Middle ethmoidal air cells	61	Cribriform plate
40	Middle concha (turbinate)	51	Perpendicular plate of ethmoidal bone	62	Middle meatus
41	Middle ear cavity	52	Dorsum sellae	63	Ostium of antrum
42	Globe	53	Superior orbital fissure	64	Infra-orbital canal
43	Posterior	ethmoidal air cells	54	Temporal lobe	65	Frontozygomatic suture
44	Anterior		55	Anterior clinoid process	66	Lesser wing of sphenoid
45	Inferior orbital fissure	56	Optic canal	67	Planum sphenoidale
46	Greater wing of sphenoid	57	Frontal sinus	68	Foramen lacerum
47	Lamina papyracea	58	Crista galli		

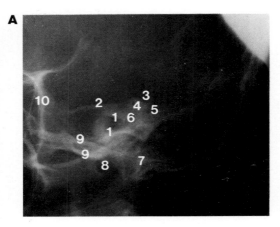

A Petrous temporal bone. Postero-anterior oblique projection

1	Internal acoustic meatus
2	Petrous part } of temporal bone
3	Arcuate eminence
4	Superior semicircular canal
5	Aditus to mastoid antrum
6	Vestibular part of inner ear
7	Mandibular condyle
8	External acoustic meatus
9	Zygomatic arch
10	Orbital margin
11	Helix of pinna of ear
12	Ossicles (malleus, incus)
13	Mandibular fossa
14	Temporomandibular joint
15	Tip of mastoid process
16	Lateral sinus
17	Styloid process
18	Mastoid air cells

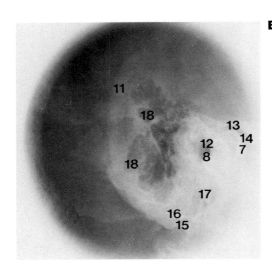

B Mastoid process. Lateral oblique projection

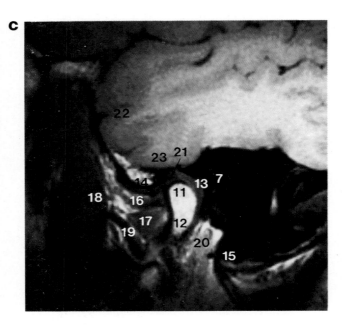

C Temporomandibular joint. Sagittal MR image (T$_1$-weighted)

Radiographs of the temporomandibular joint, **D** closed, **E** open

1	Mandibular fossa	13	Tympanic part } of temporal bone
2	Greater wing of sphenoid	14	Articular tubercle
3	Zygomatic process of temporal bone	15	Mastoid process
4	Mandibular condyle	16	Upper head } of lateral pterygoid muscle
5	Posterior border of ramus of mandible	17	Lower head
6	Malleus	18	Masseter muscle
7	External acoustic meatus	19	Deep temporal artery
8	Sinus plate	20	Parotid gland
9	Tegmen tympani	21	Articular disc
10	Pinna of ear	22	Middle } temporal gyrus
11	Head } of mandible	23	Inferior
12	Neck		

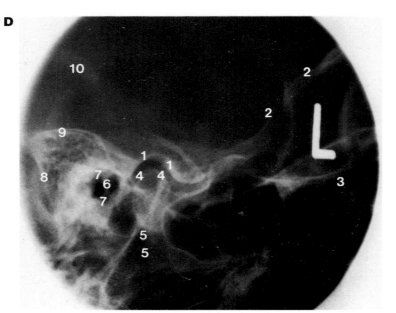

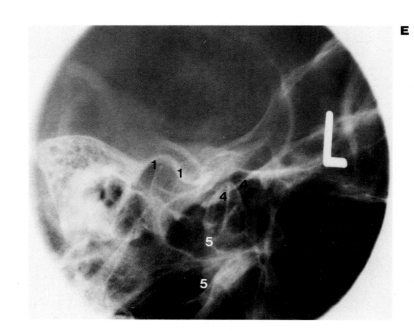

A

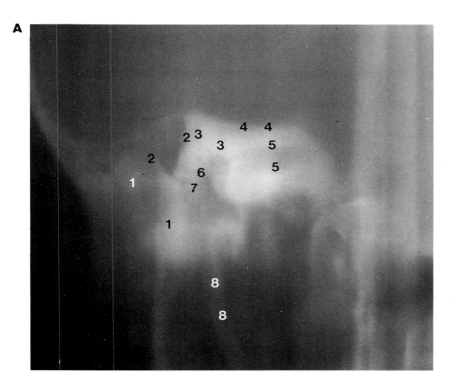

A Temporal bone. Tomogram at level of internal acoustic meatus

1	External acoustic meatus	6	Incus
2	Mastoid antrum	7	Malleus
3	Superior semicircular canal	8	Styloid process of temporal bone
4	Petrous part of temporal bone	9	Cochlea
5	Internal acoustic meatus	10	Carotid canal

B

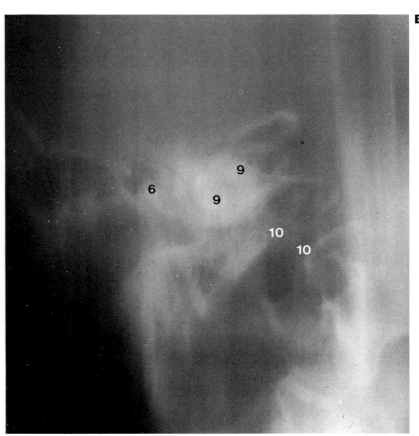

B Temporal bone. Tomogram at level of cochlea (image taken several millimetres anterior to section shown in **A**)

C CT air meatogram

This image was obtained following the injection of 4 cm³ of air into the subarachnoid space via a lumbar puncture. The patient initially sits upright and then, after the injection of air, is repositioned to lie laterally on the scan table, with the symptomatic ear uppermost. Thin axial sections are then obtained through the cerebellopontine angle, which is outlined by air. The air should extend into the normal internal acoustic meatus (IAM) and outline its contents. MRI has now superseded this investigation.

1	Air outlining cerebellopontine angle
2	Air outlining internal acoustic canal
3	Facial nerve
4	Vestibulocochlear nerve
5	Vascular loop (usually anterior inferior cerebellar artery (AICA)
6	Epitympanum
7	Aditus to antrum
8	Mastoid antrum
9	Incudomalleolar joint
10	Mastoid air cells
11	Petrous temporal bone
12	Cochlea
13	Aerated petrous apex
14	Sphenoidal sinus
15	Temporal lobe·
16	Squamous temporal bone
17	Posteromedial tract
18	Vestibule
19	Semicircular canal
20	Cerebellar hemisphere

C

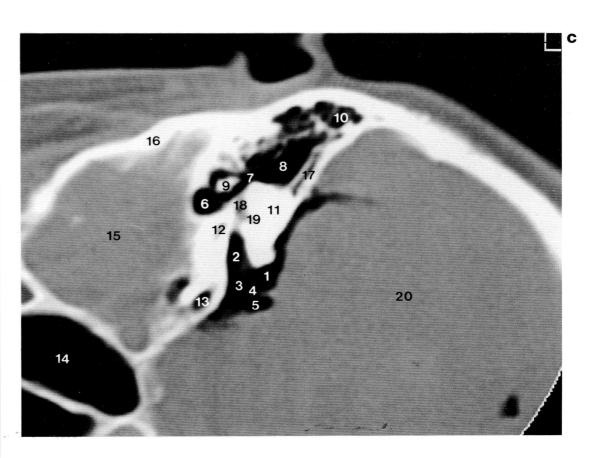

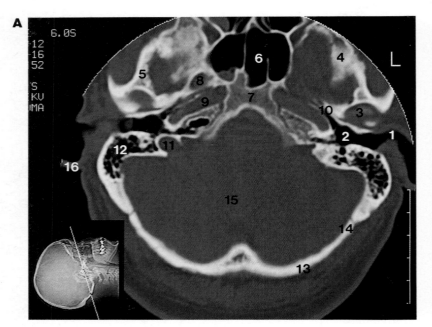

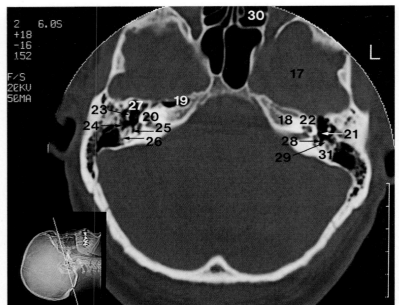

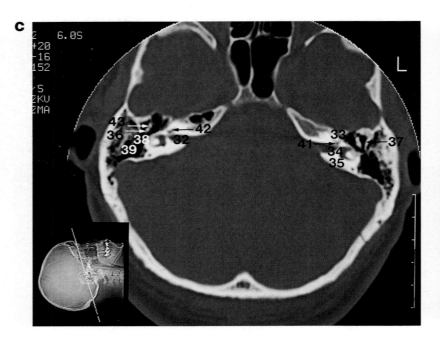

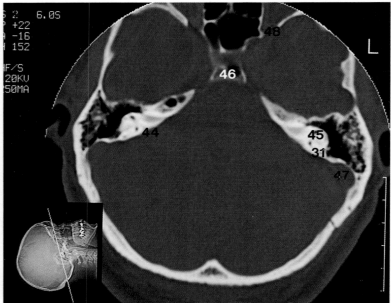

Temporal bones. Axial CT images are demonstrated at the following levels: **A** external acoustic canal; **B** cochlea; **C** internal acoustic canal and vestibule; **D** upper middle ear and mastoid

1	External acoustic meatus	12	Mastoid air cells	23	Malleus
2	External acoustic canal	13	Occipital bone	24	Facial recess
3	Temporomandibular joint	14	Lambdoid suture	25	Sinus tympani
4	Greater wing of sphenoid	15	Cerebellum	26	Horizontal portion of canal for facial nerve
5	Squamous temporal bone	16	Pinna of ear	27	Epitympanic space
6	Sphenoidal sinus	17	Temporal lobe	28	Oval window
7	Clivus	18	Petrous temporal bone	29	Pyramidal eminence
8	Foramen ovale	19	Aeration of petrous apex	30	Ethmoidal air cells
9	Carotid canal	20	Cochlea	31	Posterior semicircular canal
10	Auditory (Eustachian) tube	21	Stapes	32	Internal acoustic canal
11	Jugular foramen	22	Tensor tympani muscle	33	Geniculate ganglion

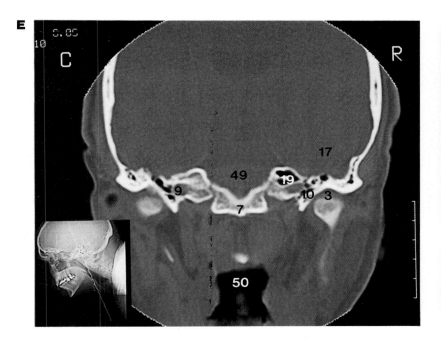
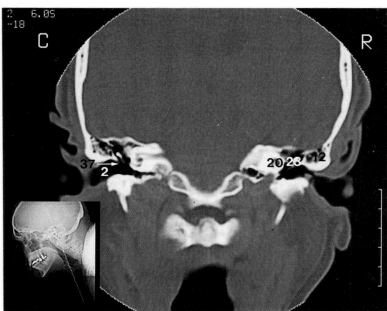

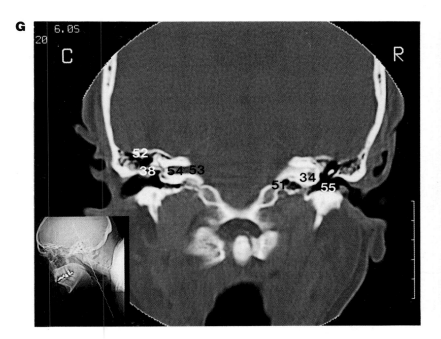
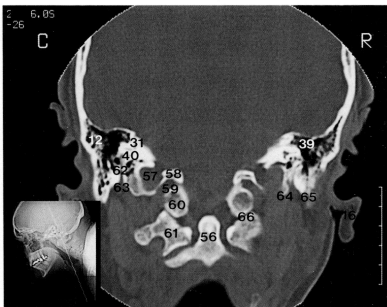

Temporal bones. Coronal CT images are demonstrated at the following levels: **E** posterior temporomandibular joint; **F** external acoustic meatus and vestibule; **G** internal acoustic meatus; **H** mastoid

34	Vestibule	45	Superior semicircular canal	56	Odontoid process (dens)
35	Vestibular aqueduct	46	Dorsum sellae	57	Jugular fossa
36	Incus	47	Sulcus of sigmoid venous sinus	58	Jugular tubercle
37	Scutum	48	Superior orbital fissure	59	Hypoglossal canal
38	Aditus to antrum	49	Brainstem	60	Occipital condyle
39	Mastoid antrum	50	Nasopharynx	61	Lateral mass of atlas (first cervical vertebra)
40	Lateral semicircular canal	51	Petro-occipital fissure	62	Descending segment of facial nerve
41	Facial nerve (first part)	52	Tegmen tympani	63	Stylomastoid foramen
42	Greater petrosal nerve	53	Internal acoustic meatus	64	Styloid process
43	Incudomalleolar joint	54	Falciform crest	65	Tip of mastoid process
44	Cochlear aqueduct	55	Middle ear cavity	66	Atlanto-occipital joint

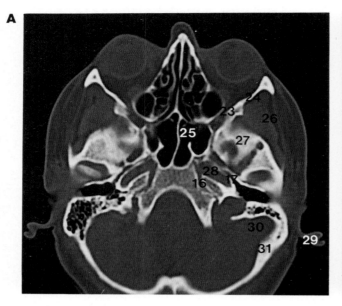 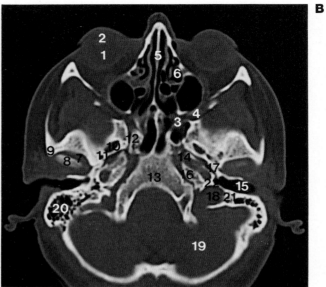

A and **B** Skull base. Axial CT images

1	Globe	12	Pterygoid (vidian) canal	23	Inferior orbital fissure
2	Lens	13	Basisphenoid	24	Greater wing of sphenoid
3	Pterygopalatine fossa	14	Foramen lacerum	25	Sphenoidal sinus
4	Pterygomaxillary fissure	15	External acoustic meatus	26	Temporalis muscle
5	Nasal septum	16	Petro-occipital fissure	27	Squamous part of temporal bone
6	Ethmoidal air cells	17	Auditory (Eustachian) tube	28	Carotid canal
7	Mandibular fossa	18	Jugular foramen	29	Pinna of ear
8	Mandibular condyle	19	Cerebellar hemisphere	30	Sulcus of sigmoid venous sinus
9	Articular condyle	20	Mastoid air cells	31	Occipital bone
10	Foramen ovale	21	Facial nerve canal		
11	Foramen spinosum	22	Caroticojugular spine		

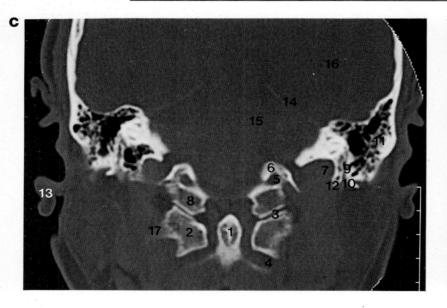 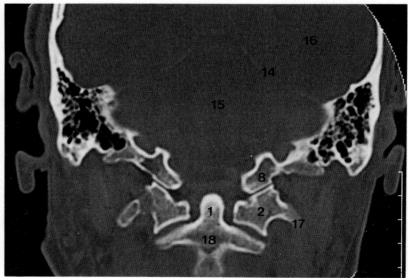

C and **D** Skull base. Coronal CT images

1	Odontoid process (dens)	7	Jugular fossa	13	Pinna of ear
2	Lateral mass of atlas (first cervical vertebra)	8	Occipital condyle	14	Tentorium cerebelli
3	Atlanto-occipital joint	9	Descending segment of canal for facial nerve	15	Posterior fossa
4	Atlanto-axial joint	10	Stylomastoid foramen	16	Cerebral hemisphere
5	Hypoglossal canal	11	Mastoid air cells	17	Transverse process of atlas
6	Jugular tubercle	12	Styloid process	18	Axis (second cervical vertebra)

A Orbital venogram

1	Frontal veins
2	Superficial connecting vein
3	Supraorbital vein
4	Angular veins
5	First ⎫
6	Second ⎬ part of superior ophthalmic vein
7	Third ⎭
8	Inferior ophthalmic vein
9	Anterior collateral vein
10	Medial collateral vein
11	Cavernous sinus
12	Internal carotid artery

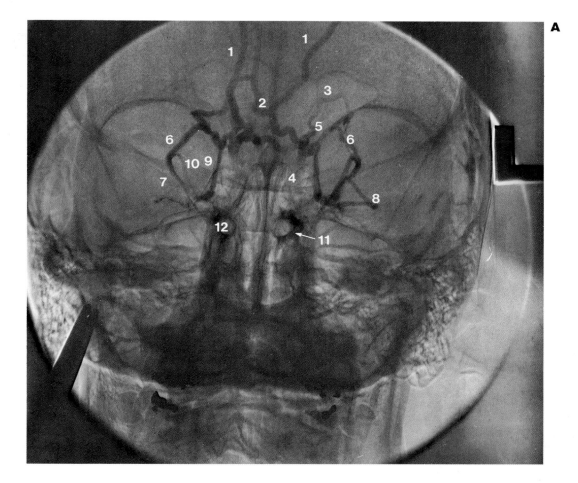

B Macrodacryocystogram

1	Lacrimal catheters
2	Site of lacrimal punctum
3	Superior canaliculus
4	Inferior canaliculus
5	Common canaliculus
6	Lacrimal sac
7	Nasolacrimal duct
8	Hard palate

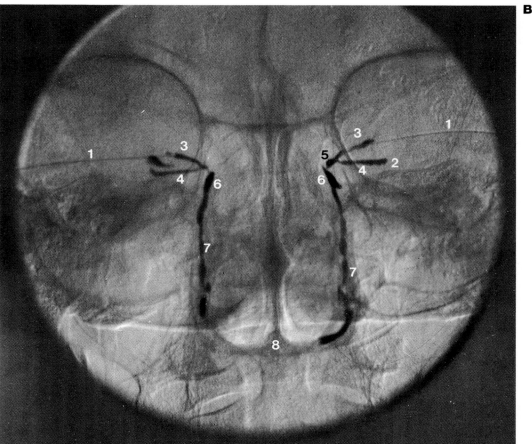

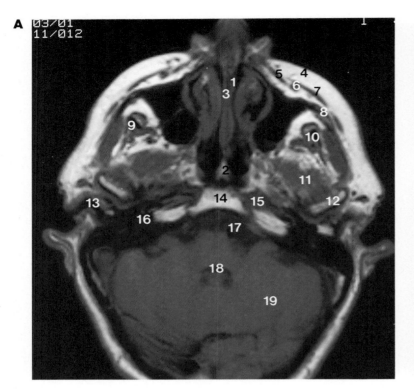

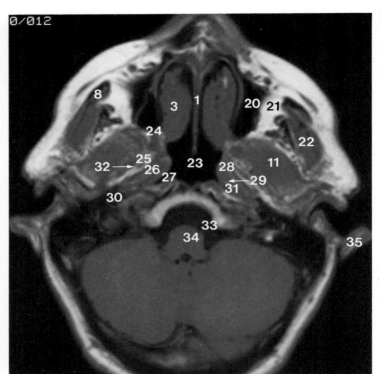

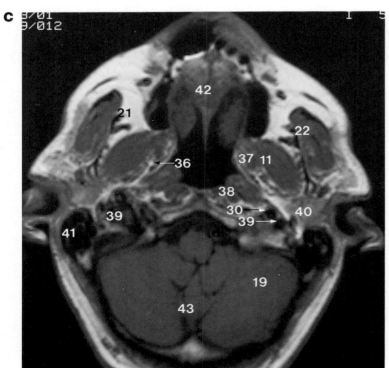

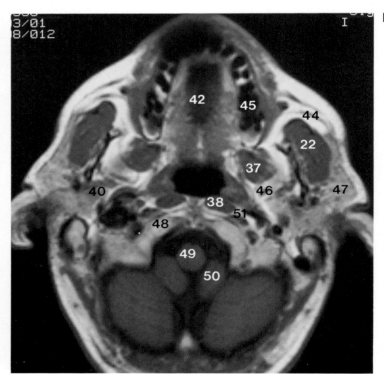

A—H Nasopharynx and oropharynx. Axial MR images (T$_1$-weighted)

1	Nasal septal cartilage	8	Zygomatic arch	16	Petrous portion of temporal	23	Nasopharynx
2	Vomer	9	Coronoid process of mandible		bone	24	Pterygomaxillary fissure
3	Inferior nasal concha	10	Temporalis muscle	17	Basilar artery	25	Pharyngobasilar fascia
4	Subcutaneous fat	11	Lateral pterygoid muscle	18	Fourth ventricle	26	Tensor veli palatini muscle
5	Levator labii superioris alaeque	12	Head of mandible	19	Left cerebellar hemisphere	27	Lateral pharyngeal recess
	nasi muscle	13	External acoustic canal	20	Maxillary sinus (antrum)	28	Pharyngeal cartilaginous end
6	Anterior facial vein	14	Marrow of clivus	21	Fat in infratemporal fossa		of auditory tube (torus
7	Zygomaticus muscle	15	Petrous apex	22	Masseter muscle		tubarius)

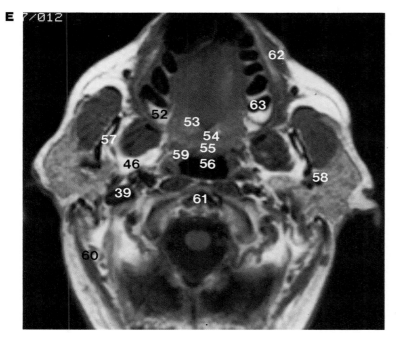

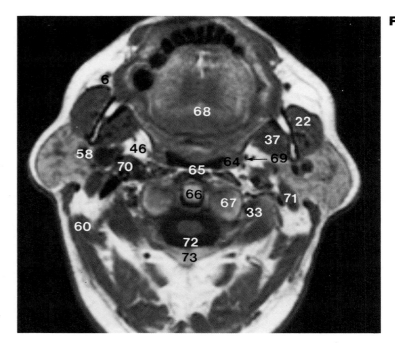

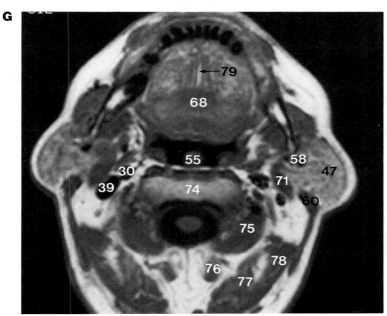

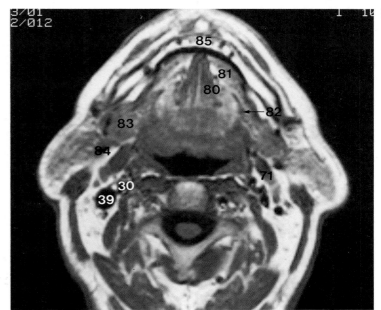

29	Auditory (Eustachian) tube	48	Occipital condyle	67	Lateral mass of atlas (first cervical vertebra)
30	Internal carotid artery	49	Spinal cord	68	Intrinsic muscles of tongue
31	Levator veli palatini muscle	50	Cerebellar tonsils	69	Ascending pharyngeal artery
32	Lateral pterygoid plate	51	Rectus capitis anterior muscle	70	Stylopharyngeus muscle
33	Vertebral artery	52	Maxillary tuberosity	71	Posterior belly of digastric muscle
34	Medulla oblongata	53	Palatine tonsils	72	Cerebrospinal fluid in subarachnoid space
35	Pinna of ear	54	Soft palate	73	Posterior arch of atlas
36	Medial pterygoid plate	55	Uvula	74	Body of axis (second cervical vertebra)
37	Medial pterygoid muscle	56	Oropharynx	75	Inferior oblique muscle
38	Longus capitus muscle	57	Ramus of mandible	76	Rectus capitis muscle
39	Internal jugular vein	58	Retromandibular vein	77	Semispinalis capitis muscle
40	Deep lobe of parotid gland	59	Palatopharyngeus muscle	78	Splenius capitis muscle
41	Mastoid process	60	Sternocleidomastoid muscle	79	Lingual septum
42	Hard palate	61	Anterior arch of atlas (first cervical vertebra)	80	Genioglossus muscle
43	Inferior cerebellar vermis	62	Buccinator muscle	81	Mylohyoid muscle
44	Parotid duct	63	Root of upper molar tooth	82	Hyoglossus muscle
45	Alveolar process of maxilla	64	Pharyngeal constrictor muscle	83	Submandibular gland
46	Parapharyngeal space	65	Posterior pharyngeal wall	84	External carotid artery
47	Parotid gland	66	Odontoid process (dens)	85	Body of mandible

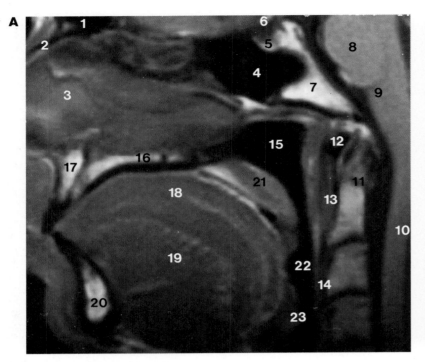
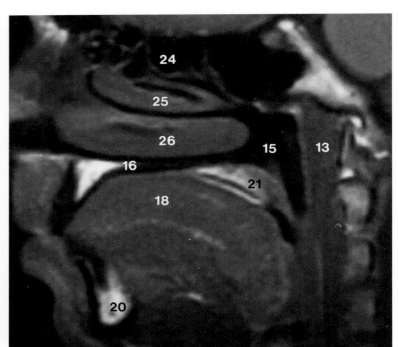
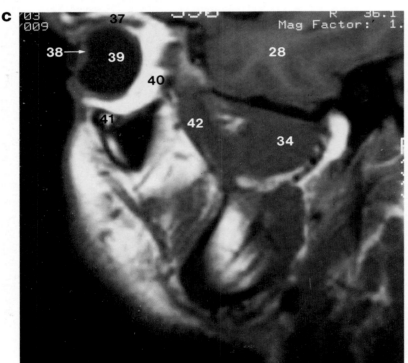
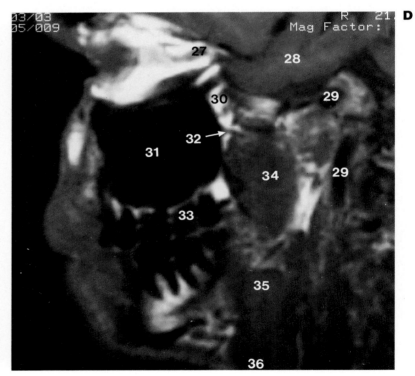

A–D Nasopharynx and oropharynx. Sagittal MR images (T_1-weighted)

1	Frontal sinus	12	Anterior arch of atlas (first cervical vertebra)
2	Nasal bone	13	Longus capitis muscle
3	Nasal septum	14	Posterior wall of pharynx
4	Sphenoidal sinus	15	Nasopharynx
5	Pituitary gland	16	Hard palate
6	Optic chiasma	17	Alveolar process of maxilla
7	Clivus	18	Tongue
8	Pons	19	Genioglossus muscle
9	Medulla oblongata	20	Mandible
10	Spinal cord	21	Soft palate
11	Odontoid process (dens)	22	Oropharynx

23	Epiglottis	34	Lateral pterygoid muscle
24	Ethmoidal air cells	35	Medial pterygoid muscle
25	Middle } nasal concha	36	Submandibular gland
26	Inferior }	37	Superior rectus muscle
27	Optic nerve	38	Lens
28	Temporal lobe	39	Globe
29	Carotid artery	40	Orbital fat
30	Pterygopalatine fossa	41	Zygoma
31	Maxillary sinus (antrum)	42	Temporalis muscle
32	Pterygomaxillary fissure		
33	Upper molar tooth		

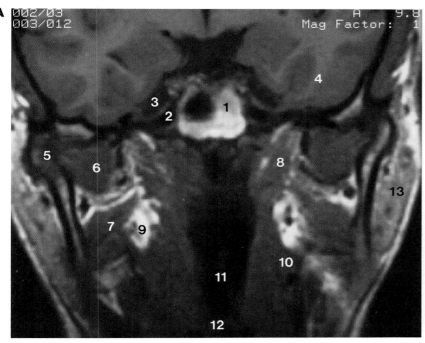
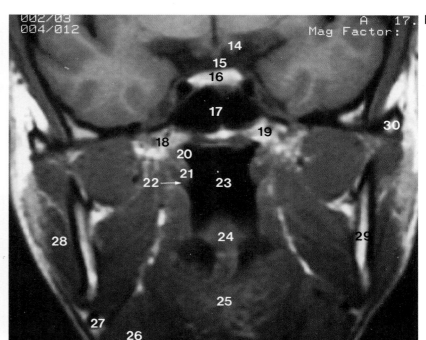
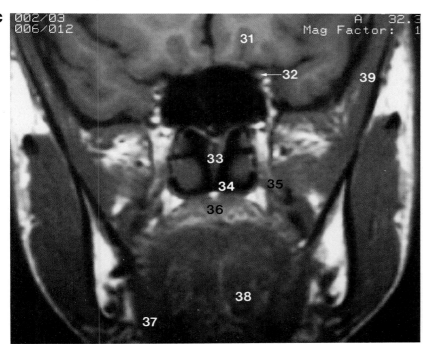
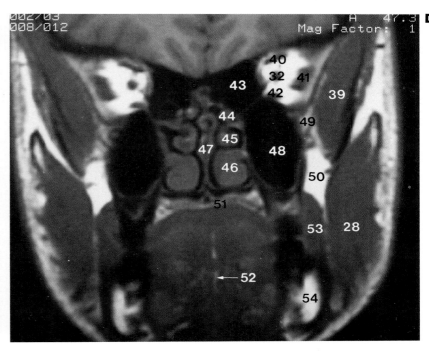

A—D Nasopharynx and oropharynx. Coronal MR images (T$_1$-weighted)

1	Clivus	14	Optic chiasma	27	Facial vessel	41	Lateral ⎫
2	Internal carotid artery	15	Pituitary stalk	28	Masseter muscle	42	Inferior ⎬ rectus muscle
3	Trigeminal ganglion	16	Dorsum sellae	29	Ramus of mandible	43	Ethmoidal air cells
4	Temporal lobe	17	Sphenoidal sinus	30	Zygomatic arch	44	Superior ⎫
5	Head of mandible	18	Greater wing of sphenoid	31	Frontal lobe	45	Middle ⎬ nasal concha (turbinate)
6	Lateral ⎫	19	Pterygoid (vidian) canal	32	Optic nerve	46	Inferior ⎭
7	Medial ⎬ pterygoid muscle	20	Lateral pharyngeal recess	33	Vomer	47	Nasal septum
8	Levator veli palatini muscle and	21	Torus tubarius	34	Nasal cavity	48	Maxillary sinus (antrum)
	tensor veli palatini muscle	22	Opening of auditory (Eustachian)	35	Pterygoid process of sphenoid	49	Infra-orbital fissure
9	Fat in parapharyngeal space		tube	36	Soft palate	50	Buccal fat pad
10	Palatal constrictor muscles	23	Nasopharynx	37	Mylohyoid muscle	51	Hard palate
11	Oropharynx	24	Uvula	38	Genioglossus muscle	52	Lingual septum
12	Epiglottis	25	Tongue	39	Temporalis muscle	53	Buccinator muscle
13	Parotid gland	26	Submandibular gland	40	Superior rectus and levator muscles	54	Body of mandible

29

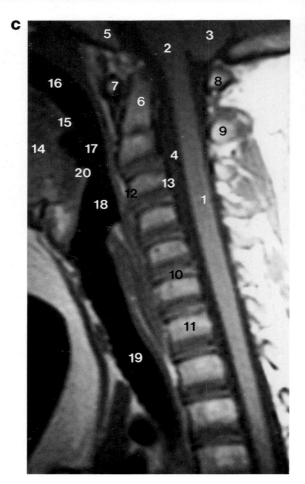

A Soft tissues of the neck. Lateral projection

1	Air in nasopharynx	10	Cricoid cartilage
2	Soft palate	11	Trachea
3	Posterior aspect of tongue	12	Thyroid cartilage
4	Retropharyngeal soft tissues	13	Vocal fold
5	Greater horn ⎫	14	Sinus of larynx
6	Body ⎭ of hyoid bone	15	Vestibular fold
7	Superior horn of thyroid cartilage	16	Vallecula
8	Cuneiform cartilage	17	Epiglottis
9	Arytenoid cartilage		

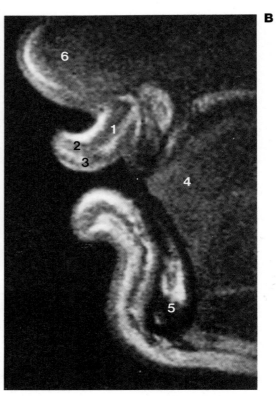

B The kiss. Sagittal MR image

1	Pars peripheralis ⎫ of orbicularis
2	Pars marginalis ⎭ oris muscle
3	Deltoid insertion of levator muscle
4	Tongue
5	Mandible
6	Nose

C Soft tissues of the neck. Sagittal MR image (T_1-weighted)

1	Spinal cord	11	Body of seventh cervical vertebra
2	Medulla oblongata	12	Anterior ⎫
3	Cerebellar tonsil	13	Posterior ⎭ longitudinal ligament
4	Cerebrospinal fluid	14	Base of tongue
5	Clivus	15	Soft palate
6	Odontoid process (dens)	16	Nasopharynx
7	Anterior arch ⎫ of atlas	17	Oropharynx
8	Posterior arch ⎭ (first cervical vertebra)	18	Hypopharynx
9	Spinous process of axis (second cervical vertebra)	19	Trachea
10	Intervertebral disc (between fifth and sixth cervical vertebrae)	20	Epiglottis

Tomography of the larynx, A at rest, B while phonating

1	Vestibule
2	Piriform fossa
3	Vestibular fold
4	Sinus of larynx
5	Vocal fold
6	Thyroid cartilage
7	Trachea

● Note how the vocal folds (5) move closer together during phonation.

A

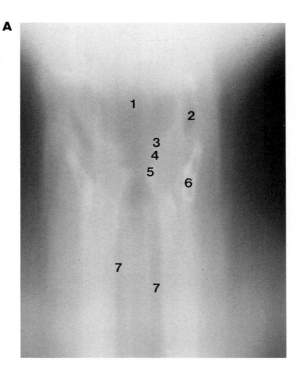

B

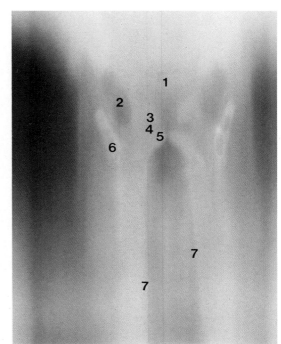

C and D Soft tissues of the neck. Coronal MR images (T$_1$-weighted)

1	Odontoid process (dens)
2	Lateral mass of atlas (first cervical vertebra)
3	Intervertebral disc (between sixth and seventh cervical vertebrae)
4	Body ⎫ of first thoracic
5	Transverse process ⎬ vertebra
6	Inferior end plate of second thoracic vertebra
7	Left vertebral artery
8	Brachial plexus
9	Scalenus medius muscle
10	Sternocleidomastoid muscle
11	Left parotid gland
12	Apex of lung
13	Trachea
14	Left lobe of thyroid gland
15	Inferior constrictor muscle
16	Brachiocephalic trunk
17	Tongue
18	Left submandibular gland
19	Body of mandible
20	Masseter muscle
21	Medial ⎫ pterygoid muscle
22	Lateral ⎭

C

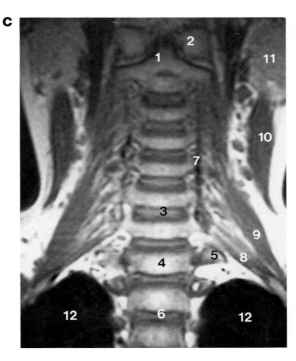

D

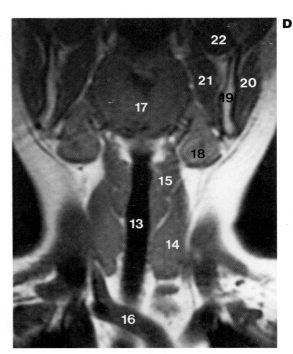

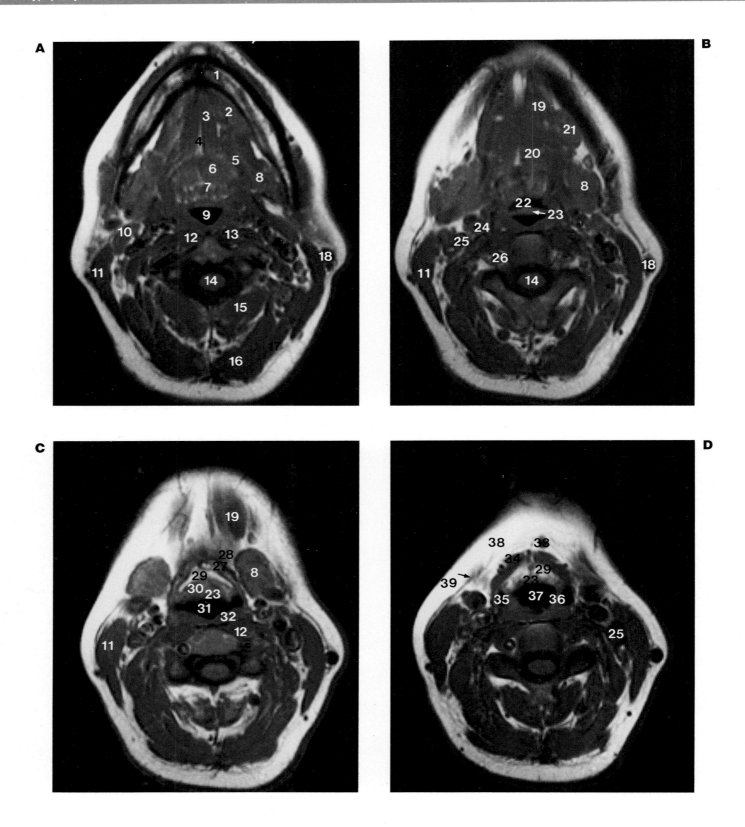

A–H Larynx and hypopharynx. Axial MR images (T$_1$-weighted)

1	Body of mandible	6	Intrinsic tongue muscle	11	Sternocleidomastoid muscle
2	Mylohyoid muscle	7	Lingual tonsils	12	Longus colli muscle
3	Genioglossus muscle	8	Submandibular gland	13	Longus capitis muscle
4	Lingual septum	9	Oropharynx	14	Spinal cord
5	Hyoglossus muscle	10	Posterior belly of digastric muscle	15	Inferior oblique muscle

E
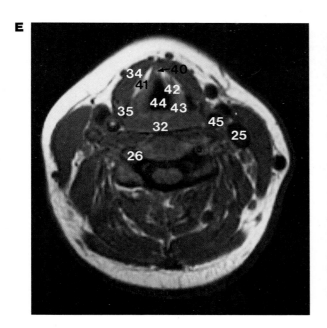

F
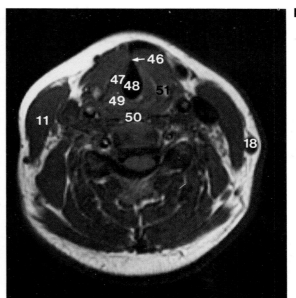

G
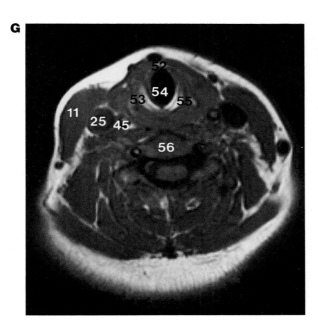

H
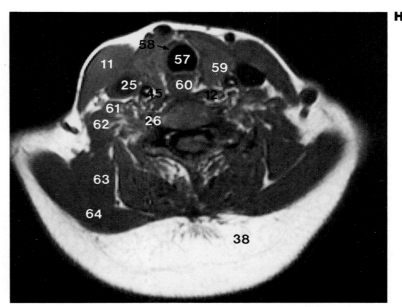

16	Semispinalis muscle	33	Anterior jugular vein	50	Prevertebral space
17	Splenius capitis muscle	34	Infrahyoid muscle	51	Inferior horn of thryoid cartilage
18	External jugular vein	35	Pyriform sinus	52	Anterior margin } of cricoid cartilage
19	Anterior belly of digastric muscle	36	Pharyngo-epiglottic fold	53	Lamina } of cricoid cartilage
20	Geniohyoid muscle	37	Laryngeal inlet	54	Subglottic space
21	Sublingual gland	38	Subcutaneous fat	55	Cricothyroid joint
22	Epiglottic valleculae	39	Platysma muscle	56	Body of fifth cervical vertebra
23	Epiglottis	40	Thyroid notch	57	Trachea
24	Internal carotid artery	41	Thyroid cartilage	58	Tracheal ring
25	Internal jugular vein	42	Vestibular fold (false cord)	59	Left lobe of thyroid
26	Vertebral artery	43	Aryepiglottic fold	60	Cervical oesophagus
27	Hyoid bone	44	Laryngeal vestibule	61	Scalenus anterior muscle
28	Suprahyoid muscles	45	Common carotid artery	62	Scalenus medius and posterior muscles
29	Pre-epiglottic space	46	Anterior commissure	63	Levator scapulae muscle
30	Base of tongue and epiglottis	47	Vocal cord	64	Trapezius muscle
31	Hypopharynx	48	Glottic space		
32	Pharyngeal constrictor	49	Arytenoid cartilage		

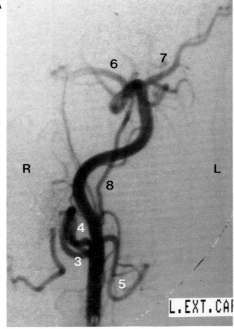

A

Digitally subtracted arteriograms of the external carotid artery, **A** anteroposterior projection, **B** lateral projection

1	Tip of catheter in external carotid artery
2	Superior thyroid artery
3	Lingual artery
4	Facial artery
5	Occipital artery
6	Maxillary artery
7	Superficial temporal artery
8	Posterior auricular artery
9	Middle meningeal artery
10	Ascending pharyngeal artery

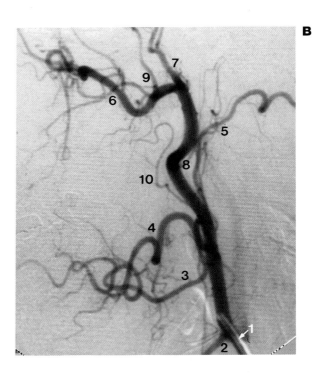

B

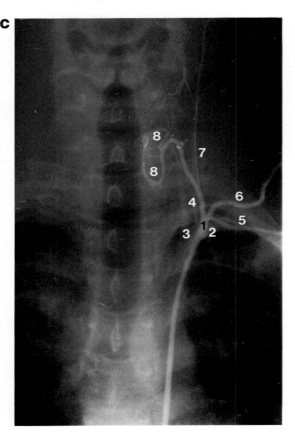

C

C Thyroid arteriogram

1	Tip of catheter in thyrocervical trunk	
2	Subclavian artery	
3	Reflux of contrast into vertebral artery	
4	Inferior thyroid artery	
5	Suprascapular artery	
6	Transverse	} cervical artery
7	Ascending	
8	Thyroid branches of inferior thyroid artery	

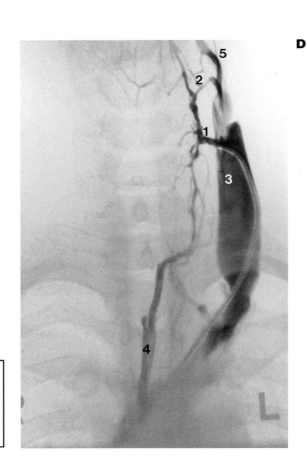

D

D Subtracted venogram of the neck

1	Tip of catheter in middle thyroid vein
2	Superior thyroid vein
3	Internal jugular vein
4	Inferior thyroid vein
5	Lingual vein

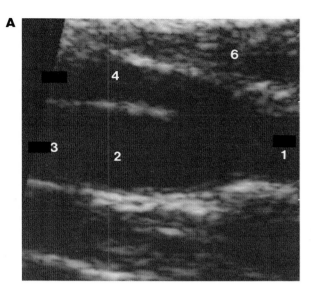

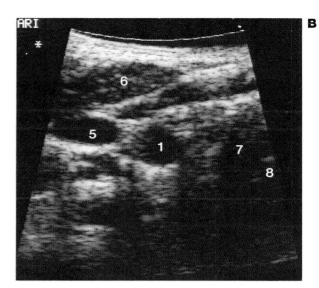

Anterior triangle of the neck. Ultrasound images A of a section along the length of the carotid sheath, B of a transverse section through the distal common carotid artery

1	Distal common carotid artery
2	Carotid bulb
3	Proximal internal ⎫
4	Proximal external ⎭ carotid artery
5	Internal jugular vein
6	Sternocleidomastoid muscle
7	Right lobe of thyroid
8	Trachea

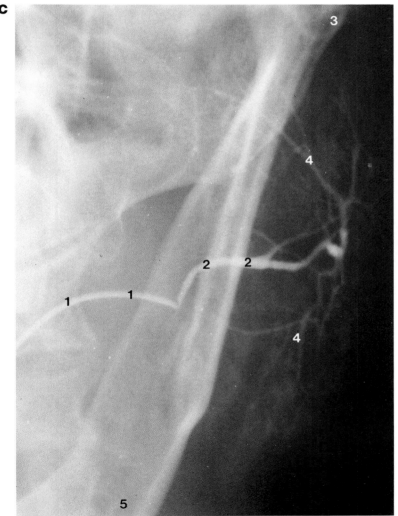

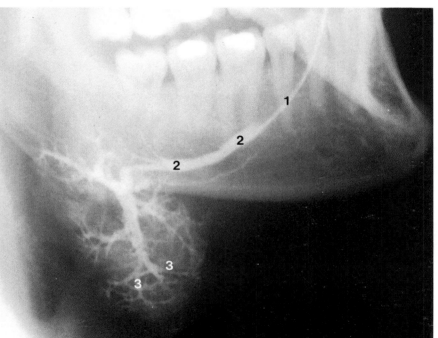

D Submandibular sialogram

1	Catheter
2	Main submandibular (Wharton's) duct
3	Secondary ductules

C Parotid sialogram

1	Catheter
2	Parotid (Stensen's) duct
3	Mastoid process
4	Secondary ductules
5	Mandible

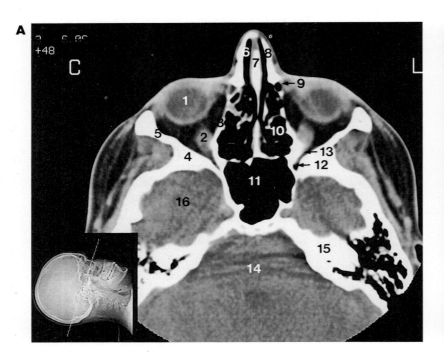
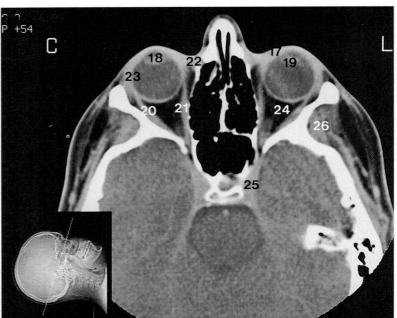
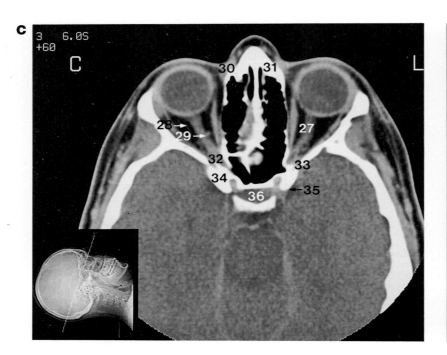
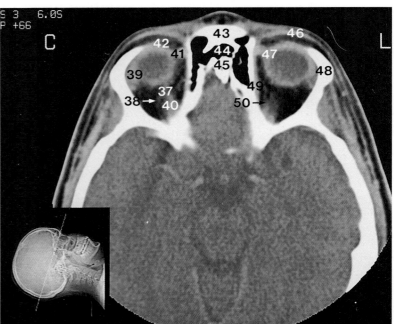

Orbits. Axial CT images are demonstrated at the following levels: **A** inferior orbit and globe; **B** mid orbit below the optic nerve; **C** mid orbit at the level of the optic nerve; **D** superior orbit.

1	Vitreous	10	Ethmoidal air cells	19	Lens	
2	Inferior rectus muscle	11	Sphenoidal sinus	20	Lateral	} rectus muscle
3	Lamina papyracea	12	Pterygopalatine fossa	21	Medial	
4	Greater wing of sphenoid	13	Inferior orbital fissure	22	Lacrimal sac	
5	Zygomatic bone	14	Brainstem	23	Sclera	
6	Nasal cavity	15	Petrous ridge	24	Retrobulbar fat	
7	Nasal septum	16	Temporal lobe	25	Cavernous sinus	
8	Nasal bone	17	Eyelid	26	Temporalis muscle	
9	Nasolacrimal duct	18	Anterior chamber	27	Optic nerve	

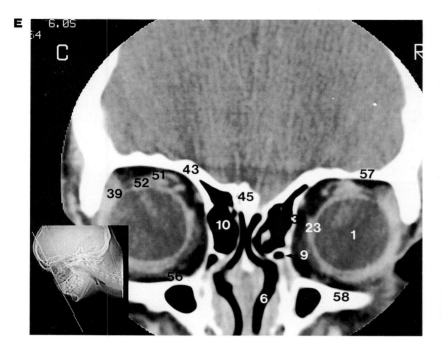

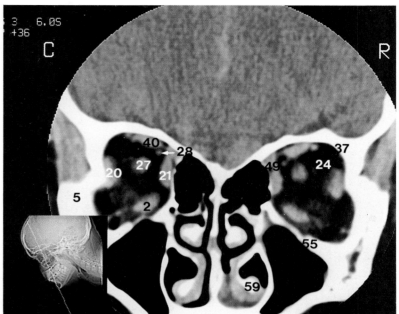

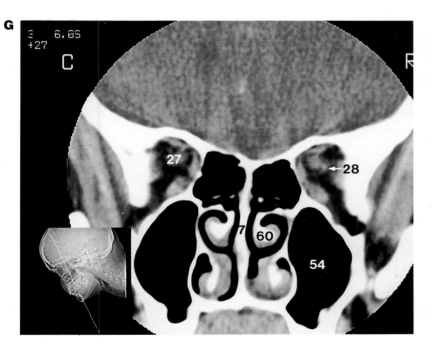

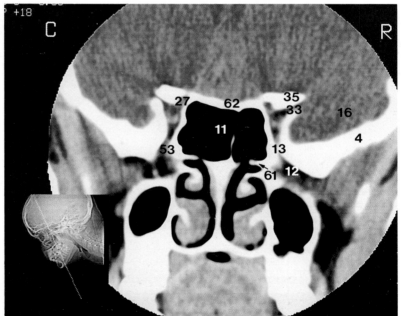

Orbits. Coronal CT images are demonstrated at the following levels: **E** globe, **F** mid orbit, **G** posterior orbit, **H** superior and inferior orbital fissures

28	Long posterior ciliary artery	40	Superior muscle group (51 and 52)	52	Superior rectus muscle	
29	Ophthalmic artery	41	Trochlea	53	Müller's muscle	
30	Angular vein	42	Orbital septum	54	Maxillary sinus (antrum)	
31	Frontal process of maxilla	43	Frontal bone	55	Infra-orbital canal	
32	Optic canal	44	Frontal sinus	56	Inferior oblique muscle	
33	Superior orbital fissure	45	Crista galli	57	Supra-orbital	} margin
34	Lesser wing of sphenoid	46	Orbicularis muscle	58	Infra-orbital	
35	Anterior clinoid process	47	Superior oblique tendon	59	Inferior	
36	Pituitary gland	48	Zygomatic process of frontal bone	60	Middle	} nasal concha (turbinate)
37	Superior ophthalmic vein	49	Superior oblique muscle	61	Superior	
38	Lacrimal vein	50	Medial ophthalmic vein	62	Planum sphenoidale	
39	Lacrimal gland	51	Levator palpebrae superioris muscle			

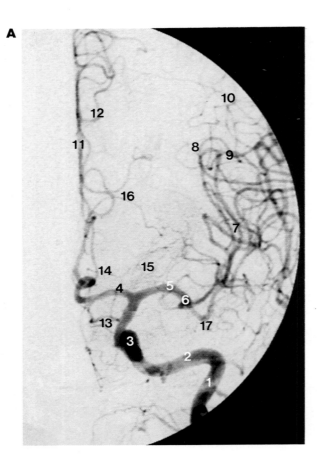

A Digitally subtracted arterial phase of carotid arteriogram. Anteroposterior projection

1	Cervical	⎫
2	Petrous	⎬ portion of internal carotid artery
3	Cavernous	⎭
4	Anterior	⎫ cerebral artery
5	Middle	⎭
6	Genu of artery	⎫ middle cerebral artery
7	Branches (in insula) of	⎭
8	Sylvian point	
9	Angular branches	⎫ of middle cerebral artery
10	Posterior parietal branches	⎭
11	Pericallosal artery	
12	Callosomarginal artery	
13	Orbitofrontal branch of pericallosal artery	
14	Recurrent artery of Heubner	
15	Lenticulostriate arteries	
16	Frontopolar artery	
17	Anterior temporal branches of middle cerebral artery	

Digitally subtracted arterial phase of carotid arteriograms. **B** lateral projection, **C** oblique projection

1	Cervical	⎫
2	Petrous	⎬ portion of internal carotid artery
3	Cavernous	⎭
4	Anterior cerebral artery	
5	Posterior communicating artery	
6	Posterior cerebral artery	
7	Anterior choroidal artery	
8	Intracranial (supraclinoid) internal carotid artery	
9	Orbitofrontal artery	
10	Frontopolar artery	
11	Pericallosal artery	
12	Callosomarginal artery	
13	Internal frontal branch of anterior cerebral artery	
14	Paracentral artery	
15	Inferior internal parietal artery	
16	Pericallosal artery extending around corpus callosum	
17	Ophthalmic artery	
18	Middle cerebral artery	
19	Operculofrontal artery	
20	Central sulcus artery	
21	Posterior parietal artery	
22	Angular artery	
23	Posterior ⎫ temporal artery	
24	Anterior ⎭	
25	Occipital artery	
26	Maxillary artery	
27	Anterior communicating artery	
28	Ethmoidal branch of ophthalmic artery	
29	Lenticulostriate artery	
30	Angular artery at Sylvian point	
31	Recurrent artery of Heubner	

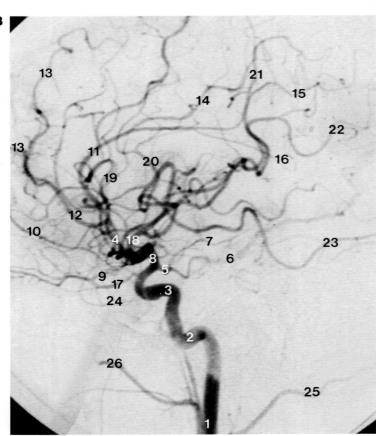

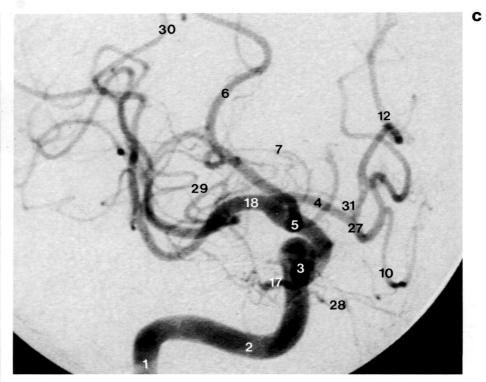

A Digitally subtracted venous phase of carotid arteriogram. Anteroposterior projection

1 Superior sagittal sinus
2 Right transverse sinus
3 Jugular bulb
4 Internal jugular vein
5 Superficial cortical veins
6 Basal vein of Rosenthal
7 Thalamostriate vein
8 Inferior sagittal sinus
9 Internal cerebral vein

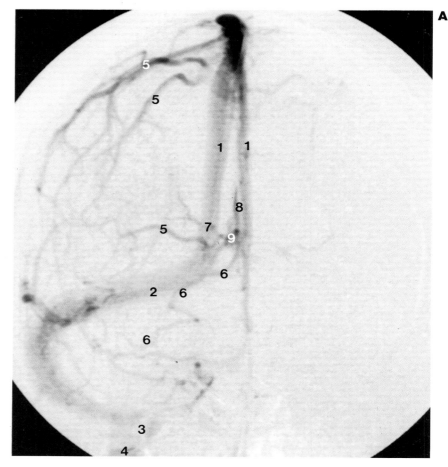

B Digitally subtracted venous phase of carotid arteriogram. Lateral projection

1   Superior sagittal sinus
2   Straight sinus
3   Inferior sagittal sinus
4   Confluence of venous sinuses (torcular Herophili)
5   Transverse sinus
6   Sigmoid sinus
7   Internal jugular vein
8   Vein of Trolard
9   Vein of Labbé
10 Superficial cerebral veins
11 Great cerebral vein of Galen
12 Basal vein of Rosenthal
13 Internal cerebral vein
14 Anterior caudate vein
15 Thalamostriate vein
16 Venous angle
17 Cavernous sinus
18 Sphenoparietal sinus

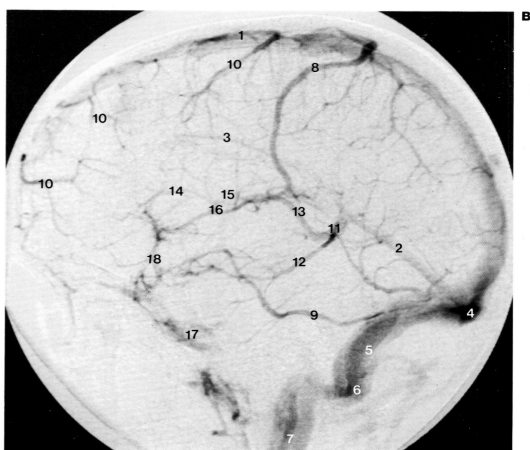

39

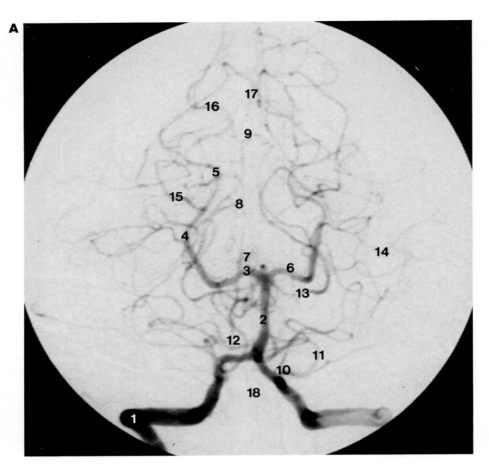

A Digitally subtracted arterial phase of vertebral arteriogram. Anteroposterior projection

 1 Vertebral artery exiting transverse foramen of atlas (first cervical vertebra)
 2 Basilar artery
 3 Posterior cerebral artery in interpeduncular cistern
 4 Posterior cerebral artery in ambient cistern
 5 Quadrigeminal portion of posterior cerebral artery
 6 Site of junction with posterior communicating artery
 7 Thalamoperforating branches of superior cerebellar artery
 8 Superior cerebellar arteries behind brainstem
 9 Vermian branch of superior cerebellar artery
10 Posterior inferior cerebellar artery
11 Medullary segment of posterior inferior cerebellar artery
12 Anterior inferior cerebellar artery
13 Superior cerebellar artery
14 Hemispheric branch of superior cerebellar artery
15 Inferior temporal artery
16 Parieto-occipital artery
17 Calcarine artery
18 Anterior spinal artery

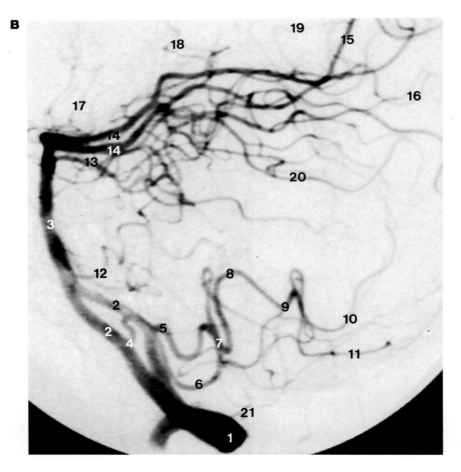

B Digitally subtracted arterial phase of vertebral arteriogram. Lateral projection

 1 Vertebral artery exiting transverse foramen of atlas (first cervical vertebra)
 2 Vertebral artery
 3 Basilar artery
 4 Origin ⎫
 5 Anterior medullary segment ⎪
 6 Lateral medullary segment ⎪
 7 Posterior medullary segment ⎬ of posterior inferior cerebellar
 8 Supratonsillar segment ⎪ artery
 9 Retrotonsillar segment ⎪
10 Inferior vermian segment ⎪
11 Hemispheric branches ⎭
12 Anterior inferior cerebellar artery
13 Superior cerebellar artery
14 Posterior cerebral artery
15 Parieto-occipital artery
16 Calcarine artery
17 Thalamoperforate ⎫
18 Posterior choroidal ⎬ branches of posterior cerebral artery
19 Splenial ⎭
20 Posterior temporal artery
21 Meningeal branch of vertebral artery

A Digitally subtracted venous phase of vertebral arteriogram. Anteroposterior projection

1	Right transverse sinus
2	Left transverse sinus
3	Straight sinus
4	Jugular bulb
5	Internal jugular vein
6	Petrosal vein
7	Superior petrosal sinus
8	Superior hemispheric vein
9	Inferior vermian vein
10	Inferior hemispheric vein
11	Anterior pontomesencephalic vein
12	Posterior mesencephalic vein

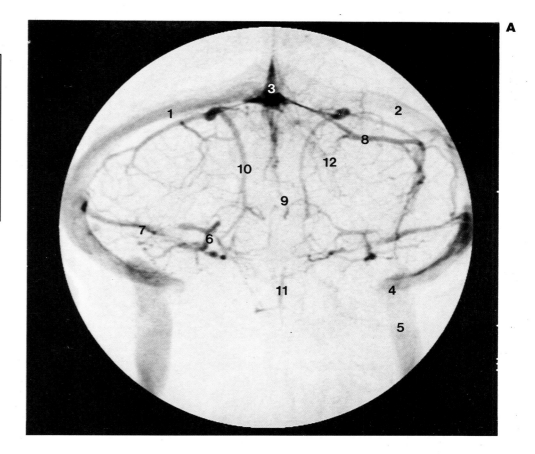

B Digitally subtracted venous phase of vertebral arteriogram. Lateral projection

1	Straight sinus
2	Great cerebral vein of Galen
3	Superior choroidal vein
4	Posterior mesencephalic vein
5	Superior hemispheric vein
6	Precentral cerebellar vein
7	Confluence of venous sinuses (torcular Herophili)
8	Inferior hemispheric vein
9	Inferior vermian vein
10	Lateral mesencephalic vein
11	Vein of the great horizontal fissure
12	Transverse sinus
13	Tonsillar vein
14	Superior vermian vein
15	Anterior pontomesencephalic vein
16	Sigmoid sinus
17	Internal jugular vein

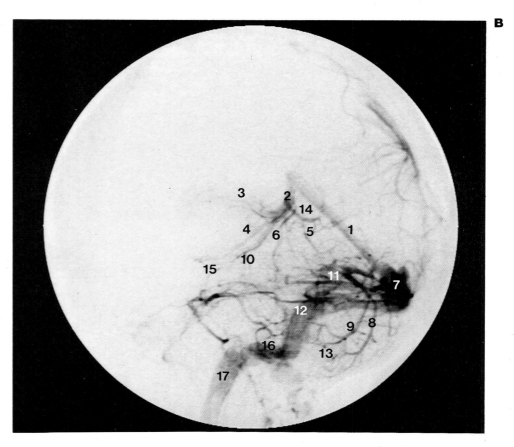

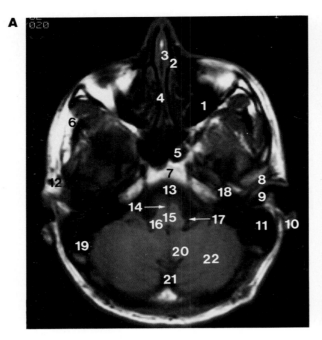
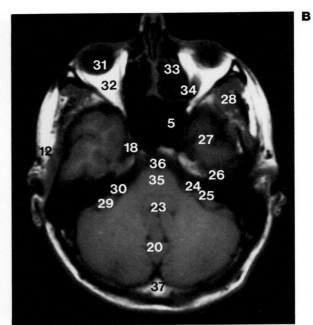
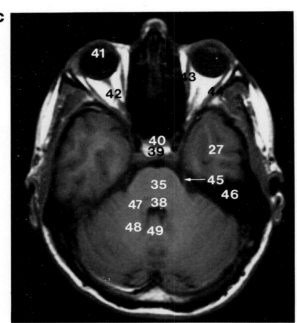
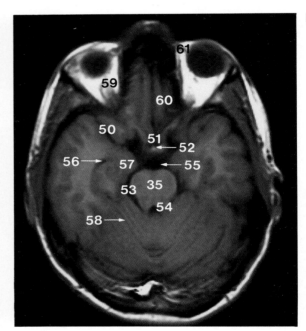

A–L Brain. Axial MR images (T$_1$-weighted)

1	Maxillary sinus (antrum)	17	Lower cranial nerve
2	Nasal cavity	18	Internal carotid artery
3	Nasal septum	19	Sigmoid sinus
4	Middle nasal concha (turbinate)	20	Inferior cerebellar vermis
5	Sphenoidal sinus	21	Cisterna magna (cerebellomedullary cistern)
6	Zygomatic arch	22	Left cerebellar hemisphere
7	Marrow of basisphenoid (clivus)	23	Fourth ventricle
8	Temporomandibular joint	24	Facial nerve
9	External acoustic meatus	25	Vestibulocochlear nerve	in internal acoustic canal
10	Pinna of ear	26	Cochlea
11	Mastoid air cells	27	Temporal lobe
12	Superficial temporal artery	28	Temporalis muscle
13	Basilar artery	29	Flocculus
14	Pyramid of medulla oblongata	30	Cerebellopontine cistern
15	Medulla oblongata		
16	Inferior cerebellar peduncle		

31	Globe	47	Middle cerebellar peduncle
32	Retro-orbital fat	48	Dentate nucleus
33	Ethmoidal air cells	49	Nodule of cerebellum
34	Inferior rectus muscle	50	Lateral sulcus (Sylvian fissure)
35	Pons	51	Optic chiasma in suprasellar cistern
36	Prepontine cistern	52	Pituitary stalk
37	Internal occipital protuberance	53	Ambient cistern
38	Tegmentum of pons	54	Superior cerebellar peduncle
39	Dorsum sellae	55	Abducent nerve
40	Pituitary gland	56	Inferior horn of lateral ventricle
41	Lens	57	Uncus
42	Optic nerve	58	Cerebellar folia
43	Medial	rectus muscle	59	Superior ophthalmic vein
44	Lateral		60	Gyrus rectus
45	Trigeminal nerve	61	Trochlea of superior oblique muscle
46	Petrous temporal bone	62	Optic tract

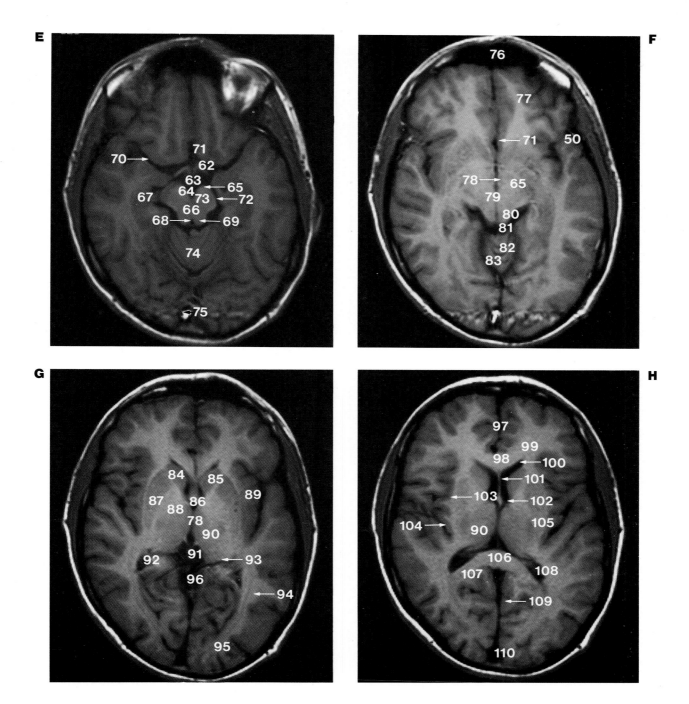

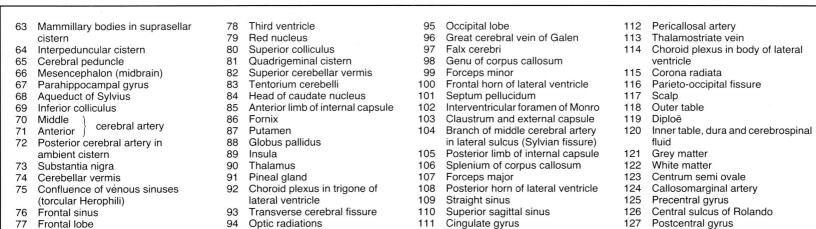

63	Mammillary bodies in suprasellar cistern	78	Third ventricle
64	Interpeduncular cistern	79	Red nucleus
65	Cerebral peduncle	80	Superior colliculus
66	Mesencephalon (midbrain)	81	Quadrigeminal cistern
67	Parahippocampal gyrus	82	Superior cerebellar vermis
68	Aqueduct of Sylvius	83	Tentorium cerebelli
69	Inferior colliculus	84	Head of caudate nucleus
70	Middle ⎫	85	Anterior limb of internal capsule
71	Anterior ⎬ cerebral artery	86	Fornix
72	Posterior cerebral artery in ambient cistern	87	Putamen
		88	Globus pallidus
73	Substantia nigra	89	Insula
74	Cerebellar vermis	90	Thalamus
75	Confluence of venous sinuses (torcular Herophili)	91	Pineal gland
		92	Choroid plexus in trigone of lateral ventricle
76	Frontal sinus	93	Transverse cerebral fissure
77	Frontal lobe	94	Optic radiations

95	Occipital lobe	112	Pericallosal artery
96	Great cerebral vein of Galen	113	Thalamostriate vein
97	Falx cerebri	114	Choroid plexus in body of lateral ventricle
98	Genu of corpus callosum		
99	Forceps minor	115	Corona radiata
100	Frontal horn of lateral ventricle	116	Parieto-occipital fissure
101	Septum pellucidum	117	Scalp
102	Interventricular foramen of Monro	118	Outer table
103	Claustrum and external capsule	119	Diploë
104	Branch of middle cerebral artery in lateral sulcus (Sylvian fissure)	120	Inner table, dura and cerebrospinal fluid
105	Posterior limb of internal capsule	121	Grey matter
106	Splenium of corpus callosum	122	White matter
107	Forceps major	123	Centrum semi ovale
108	Posterior horn of lateral ventricle	124	Callosomarginal artery
109	Straight sinus	125	Precentral gyrus
110	Superior sagittal sinus	126	Central sulcus of Rolando
111	Cingulate gyrus	127	Postcentral gyrus

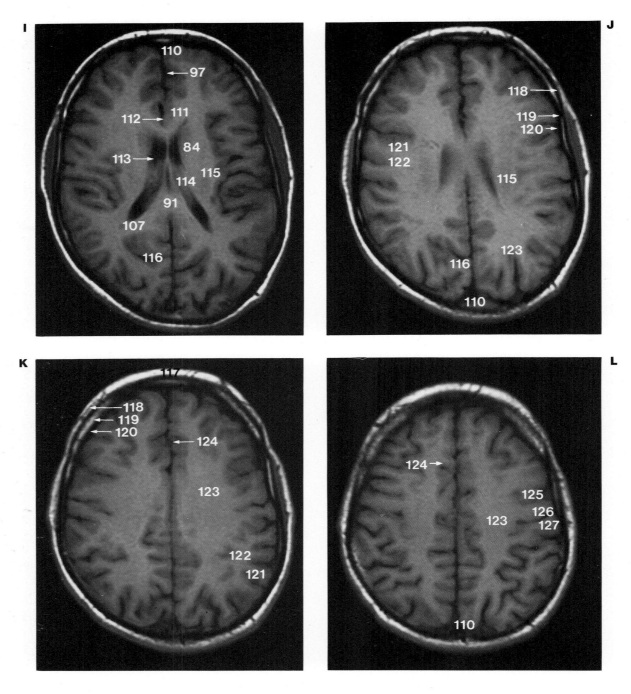

I—L Brain. Axial MR images (T$_1$-weighted)

For Key, see pp. 42–43

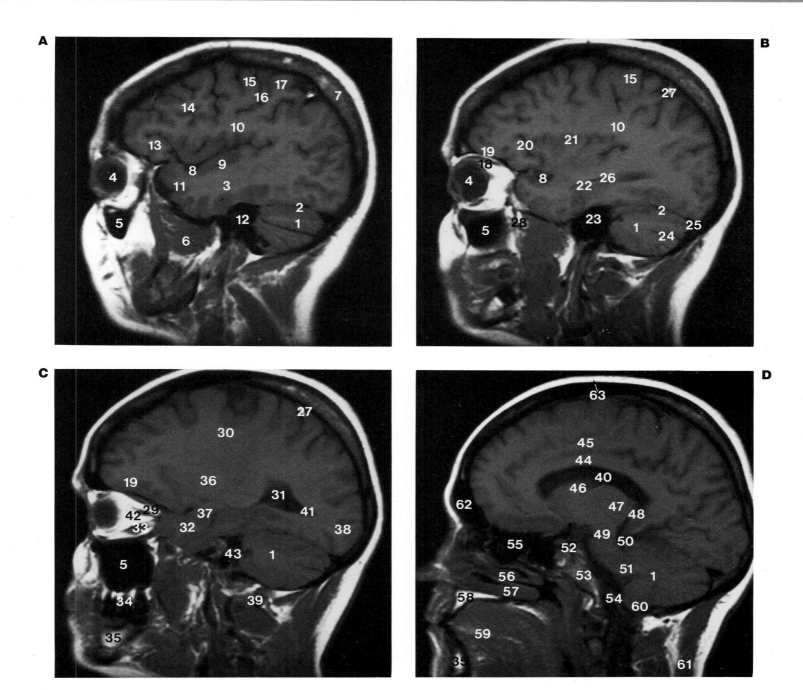

A—D Brain. Sagittal MR images (T_1-weighted)

1 Cerebellar hemisphere	17 Postcentral gyrus	32 Temporal lobe of brain	48 Fornix
2 Tentorium cerebelli	18 Superior rectus muscle	33 Inferior rectus muscle	49 Mesencephalon (midbrain)
3 Inferior longitudinal fasciculus	19 Orbital cortex of frontal lobe	34 Alveolar ridge	50 Quadrigeminal cistern
4 Globe	20 Anterior ascending ramus of	35 Mandible	51 Middle cerebellar peduncle
5 Maxillary sinus (antrum)	lateral sulcus (Sylvian fissure)	36 Lentiform nucleus	52 Internal carotid artery
6 Lateral pterygoid muscle	21 Circular sulcus of insula	37 Amygdala	53 Clivus
7 Diploë	22 Inferior horn of lateral ventricle	38 Occipital lobe	54 Basilar artery in prepontine cistern
8 Sylvian fissure	23 Internal acoustic canal	39 Vertebral artery	55 Ethmoidal air cells
9 Transverse temporal gyrus	24 Horizontal fissure of cerebellum	40 Body ⎫ of lateral	56 Middle ⎫ nasal concha
10 Superior longitudinal fasciculus	25 Transverse sinus	41 Posterior horn ⎭ ventricle	57 Inferior ⎭ (turbinate)
11 Superior temporal gyrus	26 Hippocampus	42 Retro-orbital fat	58 Hard palate
12 Petrous temporal bone	27 Cortical vein	43 Trigeminal nerve	59 Tongue
13 Inferior ⎫	28 Pterygomaxillary fissure	44 Body of corpus callosum	60 Cerebellar tonsil
14 Middle ⎭ frontal lobule	29 Optic nerve	45 Cingulate gyrus	61 Trapezius muscle
15 Precentral gyrus	30 Corona radiata	46 Head of caudate nucleus	62 Frontal sinus
16 Central sulcus	31 Trigone of lateral ventricle	47 Thalamus	63 Subcutaneous fat

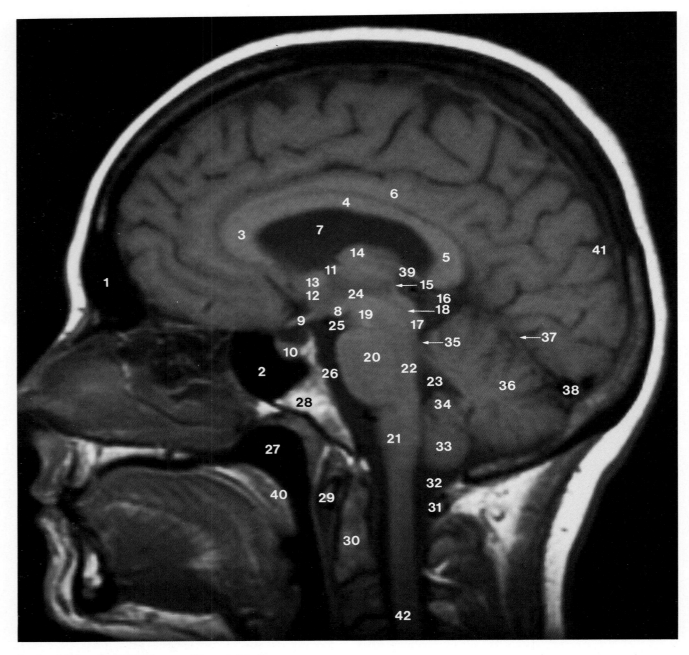

Brain. Midsagittal MR image (T$_1$-weighted)

1	Frontal sinus	16	Quadrigeminal cistern	30	Odontoid process (dens)
2	Sphenoidal sinus	17	Quadrigeminal plate of midbrain	31	Posterior arch of atlas
3	Genu	18	Aqueduct of Sylvius	32	Cisterna magna
4	Body ⎫ of corpus callosum	19	Cerebral peduncles of midbrain		(cerebellomedullary cistern)
5	Splenium ⎭	20	Pons	33	Cerebellar tonsil
6	Cingulate gyrus	21	Medulla oblongata	34	Nodule of cerebellum
7	Lateral ventricle	22	Tegmentum of pons	35	Superior medullary velum
8	Mammillary body	23	Fourth ⎫	36	Cerebellum
9	Optic chiasma in suprasellar	24	Third ⎭ ventricle	37	Tentorium cerebelli
	cistern	25	Oculomotor nerve in interpeduncular	38	Transverse sinus
10	Pituitary gland		cistern	39	Fornix
11	Interventricular foramen of Monro	26	Prepontine cistern	40	Uvula
12	Lamina terminalis	27	Nasopharynx	41	Parieto-occipital fissure
13	Anterior commissure	28	Fat in marrow of clivus	42	Cervical spinal cord
14	Massa intermedia	29	Anterior arch of atlas (first cervical		
15	Posterior commissure		vertebra)		

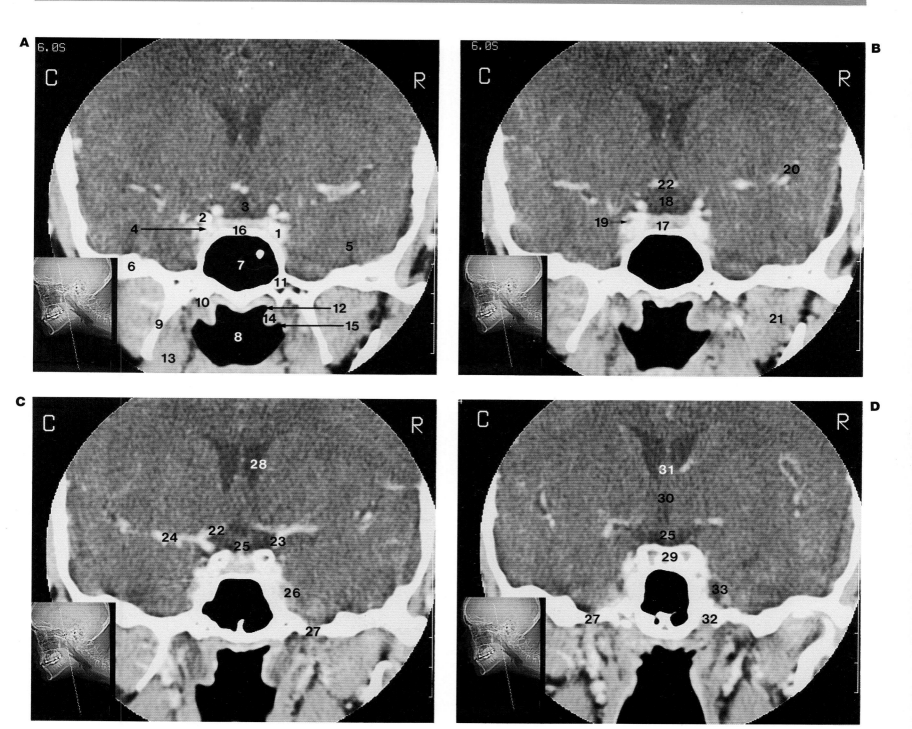

A–D Pituitary fossa (sella turcica). Coronal CT images

These images show 2 mm coronal slices through the sella turcica (pituitary fossa) from anterior (**A**) to posterior (**D**) during the intravenous infusion of non-ionic water-soluble contrast medium.

1	Cavernous sinus	12	Pharyngeal recess (fossa of Rosenmüller)	23	Supraclinoid internal carotid artery
2	Anterior clinoid process	13	Medial pterygoid muscle	24	Middle cerebral artery
3	Suprasellar cistern	14	Torus tubarius	25	Pituitary stalk
4	Cavernous carotid artery	15	Orifice of auditory (Eustachian) tube	26	Trigeminal nerve
5	Temporal lobe of brain	16	Floor of pituitary fossa (sella turcica)	27	Foramen ovale
6	Floor of middle cranial fossa	17	Pituitary gland	28	Lateral ventricle
7	Sphenoidal sinus	18	Optic chiasma	29	Dorsum sellae
8	Nasopharynx	19	Oculomotor nerve	30	Third ventricle
9	Lateral	20	Lateral sulcus (Sylvian fissure) with branches of middle	31	Body of fornix
10	Medial } pterygoid plate		cerebral artery	32	Foramen lacerum
11	Pterygoid (vidian) canal	21	Lateral pterygoid muscle	33	Trigeminal (gasserian) ganglion in recess (Meckel's cave)
		22	Anterior cerebral artery		

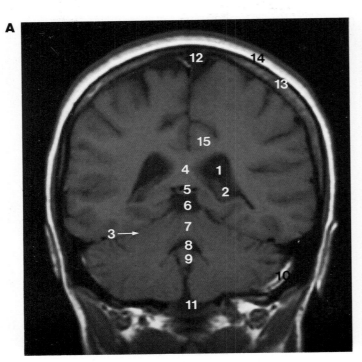
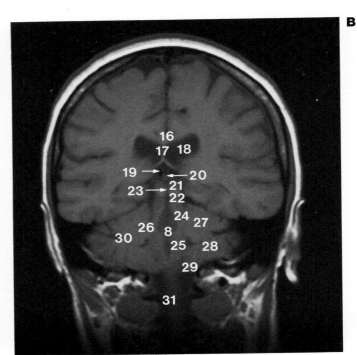
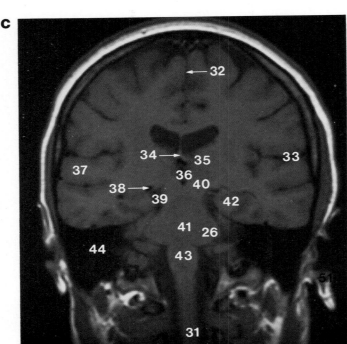
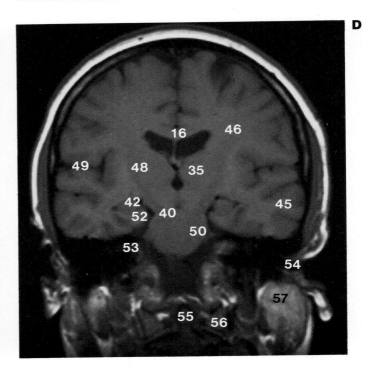

A–G Brain. Coronal MR images (T₁-weighted)

1	Trigone of lateral ventricle	16	Corpus callosum	31	Spinal cord
2	Choroid plexus	17	Septum pellucidum	32	Falx cerebri in longitudinal fissure
3	Tentorium cerebelli	18	Body of lateral ventricle	33	Lateral sulcus (Sylvian fissure)
4	Splenium of corpus callosum	19	Internal cerebral vein	34	Fornix
5	Great cerebral vein of Galen	20	Pineal gland	35	Thalamus
6	Quadrigeminal cistern	21	Superior	colliculus	36	Third ventricle
7	Superior vermis	22	Inferior		37	Superior temporal gyrus
8	Fourth ventricle	23	Aqueduct of Sylvius	38	Posterior cerebral artery
9	Nodule of cerebellum	24	Superior	cerebellar peduncle	39	Ambient cistern
10	Sigmoid sinus	25	Inferior		40	Cerebral peduncle
11	Cisterna magna (cerebellomedullary cistern)	26	Middle		41	Pons
12	Superior sagittal sinus	27	Superior	cerebellar hemisphere	42	Hippocampus
13	Diploë	28	Inferior		43	Medulla oblongata
14	Subcutaneous fat	29	Cerebellar tonsil	44	Petrous temporal bone
15	Cingulate gyrus	30	Horizontal cerebellar fissure	45	Grey matter

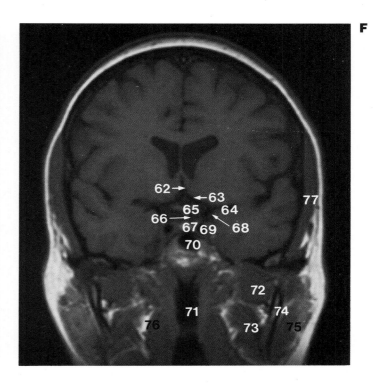

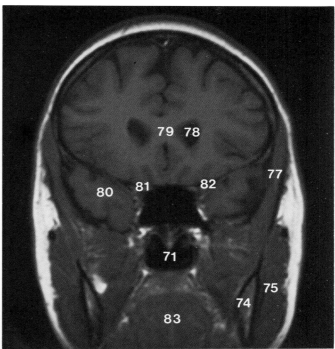

46 Corona radiata
47 Insula
48 Internal capsule
49 Branch of middle cerebral artery in lateral sulcus (Sylvian fissure)
50 Longitudinal pontine bundle in pons
51 Pinna of ear
52 Parahippocampal gyrus
53 Facial and vestibulocochlear nerves in internal acoustic meatus
54 External acoustic meatus
55 Odontoid process (dens)
56 Atlas (first cervical vertebra)
57 Parotid gland
58 Head of caudate nucleus
59 Interpeduncular cistern
60 Inferior horn of lateral ventricle
61 Clivus
62 Interhemispheric cistern
63 Anterior ⎱
64 Middle ⎰ cerebral artery
65 Optic chiasma in suprasellar cistern
66 Pituitary stalk in suprasellar cistern
67 Dorsum sellae
68 Supraclinoid ⎱ internal carotid
69 Intracavernous ⎰ artery
70 Sphenoidal sinus
71 Nasopharynx
72 Lateral ⎱
73 Medial ⎰ pterygoid muscle
74 Mandible
75 Masseter muscle
76 Fat in parapharyngeal space
77 Temporalis muscle
78 Anterior horn of lateral ventricle
79 Genu of corpus callosum
80 Temporal lobe of cerebrum
81 Optic nerve
82 Anterior clinoid process
83 Tongue

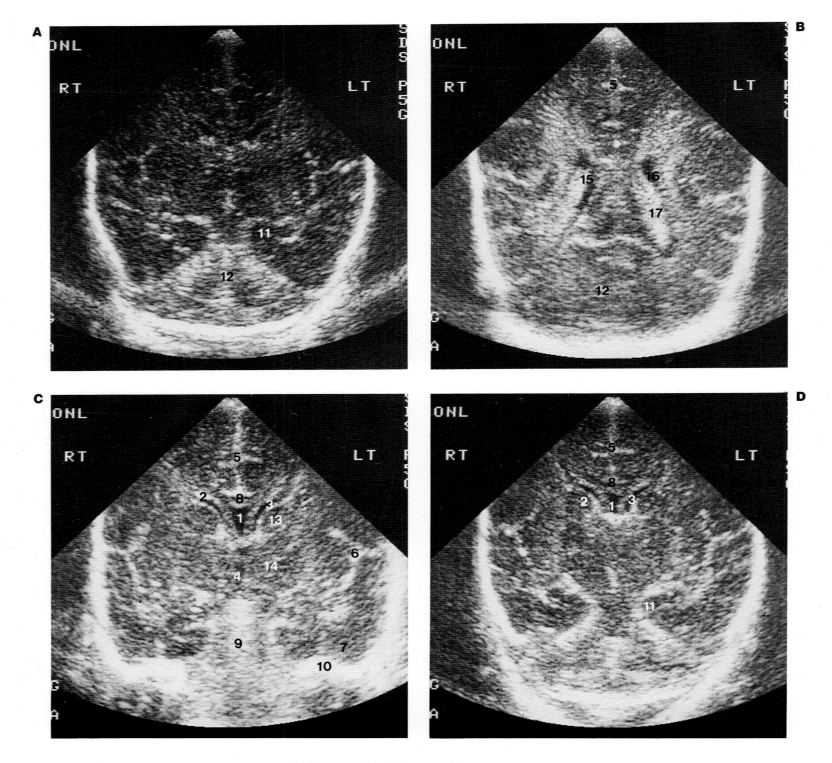

Neonatal brain. A—D coronal ultrasound images, E—H parasagittal ultrasound images

1	Cavum septum pellucidum	10	Greater wing of sphenoid	19	Quadrigeminal cistern
2	Anterior horn of right	11	Hippocampal gyrus	20	Brainstem
3	Anterior horn of left } lateral ventricle	12	Cerebellum	21	Clivus
4	Third ventricle	13	Left caudate nucleus	22	Pituitary fossa (sella turcica)
5	Interhemispheric fissure	14	Thalamus	23	Parasagittal sulci and gyri
6	Left Sylvian fissure	15	Body of right	24	Posterior horn of right
7	Left temporal lobe	16	Body of left } lateral ventricle	25	Posterior horn of left } lateral ventricle
8	Corpus callosum	17	Choroid plexus in left lateral ventricle	26	Orbital roof
9	Ethmoidal complex	18	Fourth ventricle	27	Posterior rim of foramen magnum

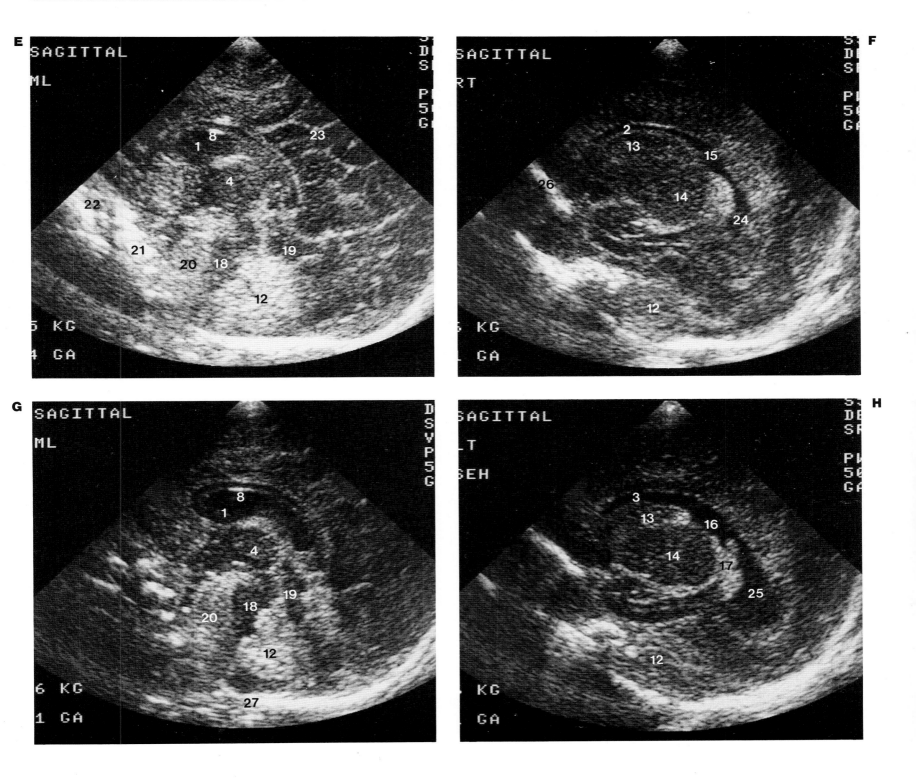

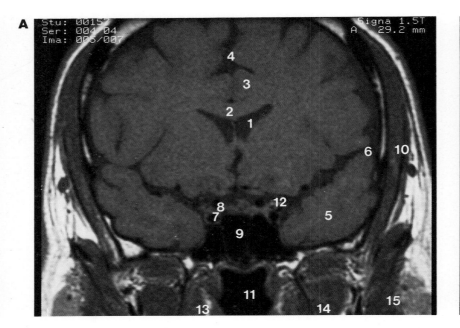
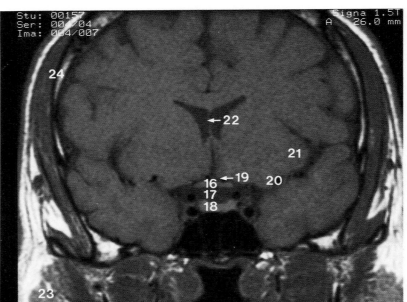
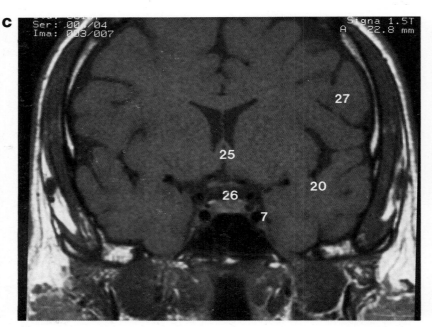
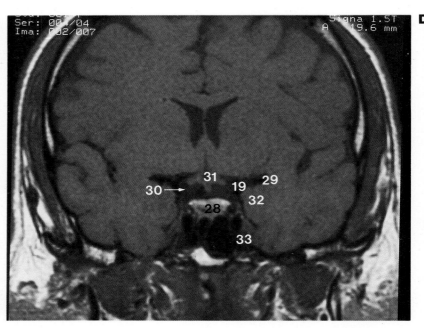

Pituitary fossa (sella turcica). Coronal MR images (T$_1$-weighted). A at the level of the anterior clinoid, **B** mid fossa, **C** at the level of the pituitary stalk, **D** at the level of the dorsum sellae

1	Anterior horn of lateral ventricle	12	Anterior clinoid process	23	Parotid gland
2	Corpus callosum	13	Medial ⎫	24	Parietal bone
3	Cingulate gyrus	14	Lateral ⎬ pterygoid muscle	25	Interhemispheric cistern
4	Interhemispheric fissure	15	Masseter muscle	26	Pituitary stalk
5	Temporal lobe of brain	16	Optic chiasma	27	Parietal lobe of brain
6	Lateral sulcus (Sylvian fissure)	17	Suprasellar cistern	28	Dorsum sellae
7	Internal carotid artery in cavernous sinus	18	Pituitary gland	29	Middle cerebral artery
8	Supraclinoid internal carotid artery	19	Anterior cerebral artery	30	Bifurcation of internal carotid artery
9	Sphenoidal sinus	20	Branch of middle cerebral artery in lateral sulcus (Sylvian fissure)	31	Third ventricle
10	Temporalis muscle	21	Insula	32	Uncus
11	Nasopharynx	22	Septum pellucidum	33	Trigeminal (gasserian) ganglion

Vertebral column and spinal cord

A Cervical spine. Anteroposterior projection

B Dried cervical vertebra. Anteroposterior projection

1	Region of vocal cords
2	Trachea
3	Posterolateral lip (uncus)
4	Superior articular process (facet)
5	Posterior tubercle ⎫
6	Intertubercular lamella ⎬ of transverse process
7	Inferior articular process (facet)
8	Body
9	Spinous process

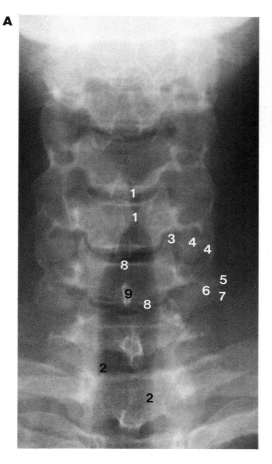

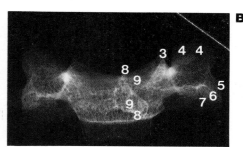

C Cervical spine. Lateral projection

D Dried atlas (first cervical vertebra). Lateral projection

E Dried axis (second cervical vertebra). Lateral projection

F Dried fourth cervical vertebra. Lateral projection

1	Anterior arch ⎫ of atlas (first cervical vertebra)
2	Spinous process ⎬
3	Odontoid process (dens) ⎫ of axis (second
4	Body ⎬ cervical vertebra)
5	Spinous process ⎭
6	Superior articular process (facet) ⎫
7	Anterior tubercle of transverse process ⎪ of fourth
8	Posterior tubercle of transverse process ⎬ cervical
9	Inferior articular process (facet) ⎪ vertebra
10	Spinous process ⎭

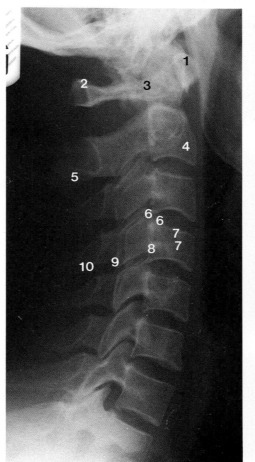

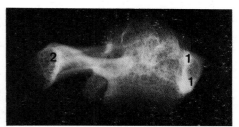

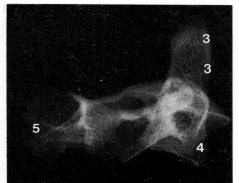

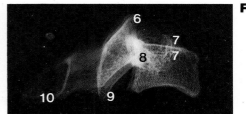

53

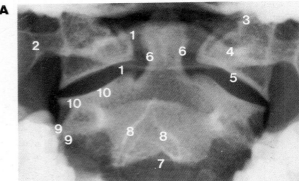

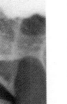

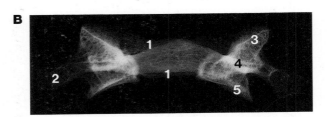

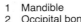

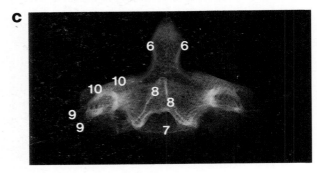

A Atlas (first cervical vetrebra) and axis (second cervical vertebra). 'Open-mouth' anteroposterior projection

B Dried atlas (first cervical vertebra). Anteroposterior projection

C Dried axis (second cervical vertebra). Anteroposterior projection

D Cervical spine of a 3-year-old child. Lateral projection

● The apparent widening of the atlanto-axial joint (11) is a normal feature at this age.

1	Anterior arch		of atlas (first cervical vertebra)
2	Transverse process		
3	Superior articular process (facet)		
4	Lateral mass		
5	Inferior articular process (facet)		
6	Odontoid process (dens)		of axis (second cervical vertebra)
7	Body		
8	Bifid spinous process		
9	Transverse process		
10	Superior articular process (facet)		
11	Atlanto-axial joint		

E Cervical spine. Oblique projection

1	Mandible	10	Intervertebral foramen
2	Occipital bone	11	Trachea
3	Hyoid bone	12	Left
4	Transverse process	13	Right ⎱ first rib
5	Posterior tubercle of transverse process		
6	Body		of fifth cervical vertebra
7	Posterolateral lip (uncus)		
8	Lamina		
9	Spinous process		

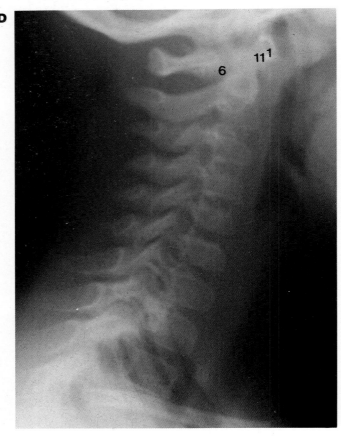

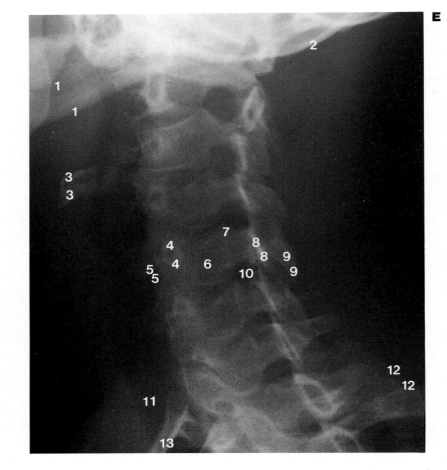

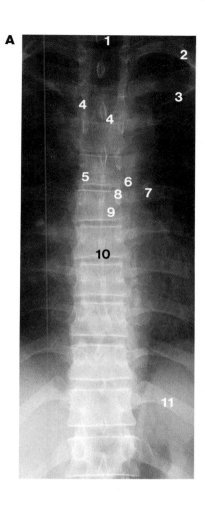

A **Thoracic spine. Anteroposterior projection**

B **Dried thoracic vertebra. Anteroposterior projection**

C **Thoracic spine. Lateral projection**

D **Dried sixth thoracic vertebra. Lateral projection**

Thoracic spine, **E** of a 7-day-old neonate, **F** of a 12-year-old child. Lateral projections

1	First thoracic vertebra
2	First rib
3	Clavicle
4	Trachea
5	Right ⎫ main bronchus
6	Left ⎭
7	Transverse process ⎫
8	Pedicle ⎪ of sixth thoracic
9	Body ⎬ vertebra
10	Spinous process ⎭
11	Ribs
12	Superior articular process (facet)
13	Transverse process
14	Spinous process
15	Inferior articular process (facet)
16	Inferior vertebral notch
17	Body
18	Pedicle
19	Site of intervertebral disc
20	Superior ⎫ annular epiphysial
21	Inferior ⎭ discs for vertebral body

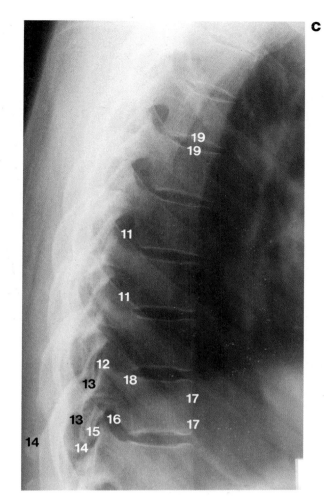

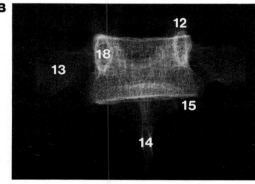

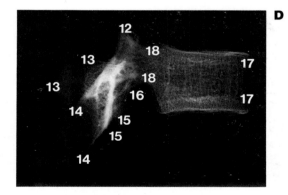

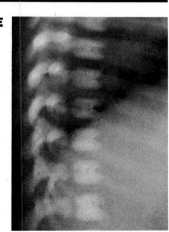

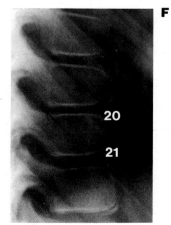

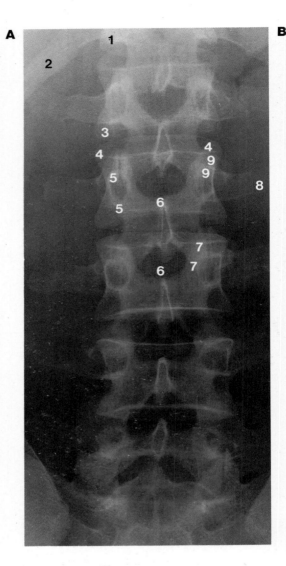

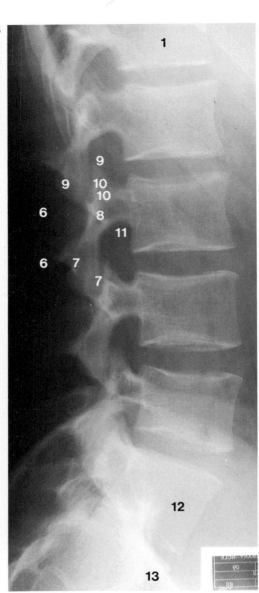

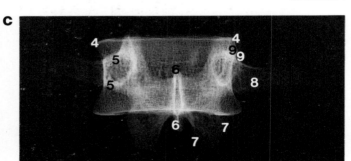

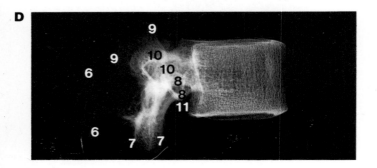

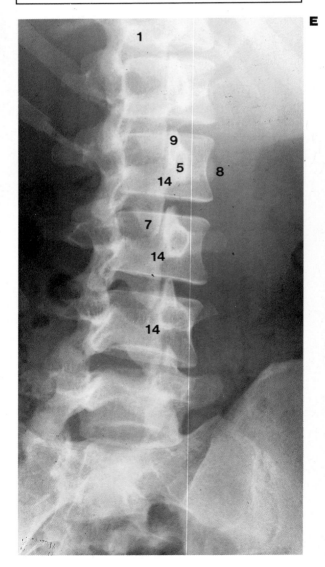

A Lumbar spine. Anteroposterior radiograph

B Lumbar spine. Lateral projection

C Dried second lumbar vertebra. Anteroposterior projection

D Dried second lumbar vertebra. Lateral projection

E Lumbar spine. Oblique projection

1	Body of twelfth thoracic vertebra
2	Right twelfth rib
3	Body of first lumbar vertebra
4	Body
5	Pedicle
6	Spinous process
7	Inferior articular process (facet)
8	Transverse process
9	Superior articular process (facet)
10	Mamillary process
11	Inferior vertebral notch
12	Fifth lumbar vertebra
13	Sacral promontory
14	Pars interarticularis

of second lumbar vertebra

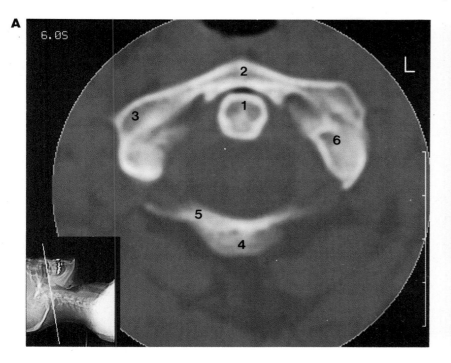

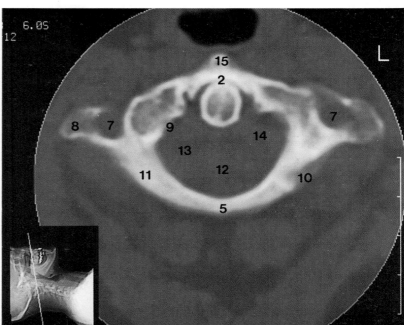

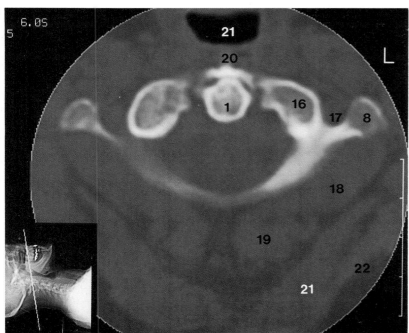

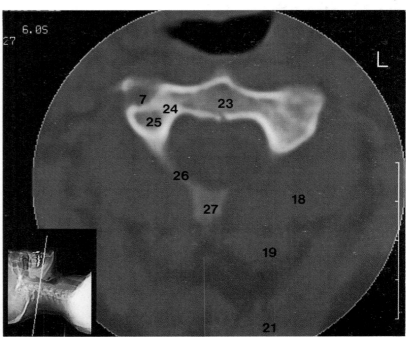

A—D Cervical spine. Axial CT images at the level of the atlas (first cervical vertebra)

1	Odontoid process (dens)		10	Groove for vertebral artery	19	Rectus capitis muscle
2	Anterior arch		11	Lamina	20	Prevertebral soft tissue
3	Lateral mass		12	Spinal cord	21	Semispinalis capitis muscle
4	Spinous process	of atlas (first cervical vertebra)	13	Subarachnoid space	22	Splenius capitis muscle
5	Posterior arch		14	Epidural space	23	Body of axis (second cervical vertebra)
6	Superior articular process (facet)		15	Anterior tubercle of atlas	24	Pedicle
7	Transverse foramen		16	Inferior articular process (facet)	25	Articular pillar
8	Transverse process		17	Vertebral artery in transverse foramen	26	Lamina
9	Attachment of transverse ligament		18	Inferior oblique muscle	27	Spinous process of axis

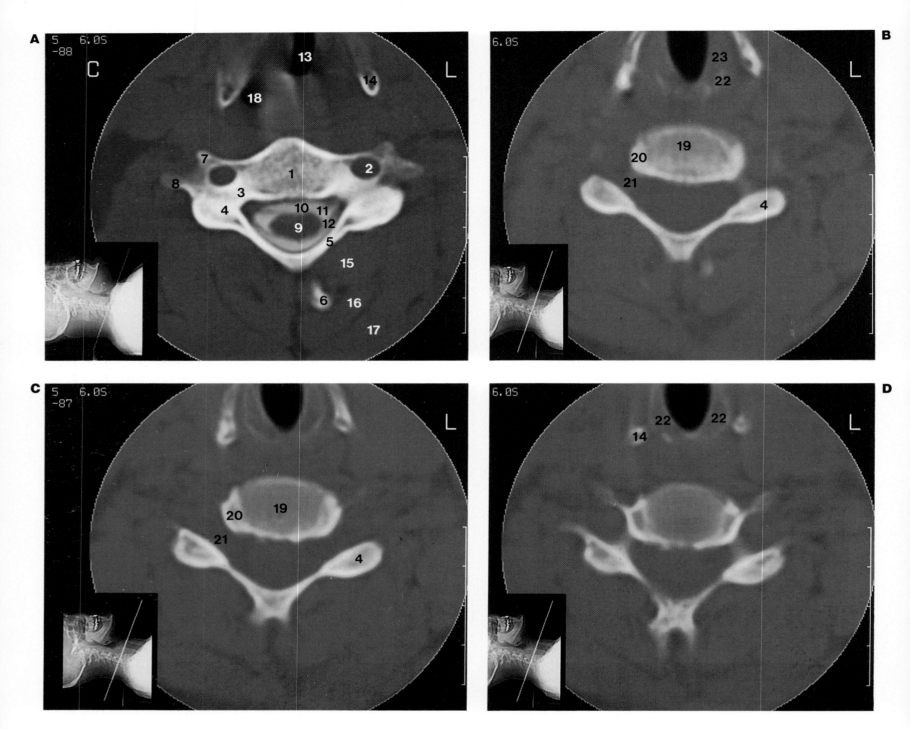

A–D Cervical spine. Axial CT images at the level of the fifth and sixth cervical vertebrae

1	Body of fifth cervical vertebra	9	Spinal cord	17	Semispinalis capitis muscle
2	Transverse foramen	10	Contrast medium in subarachnoid space	18	Pyriform sinus
3	Pedicle	11	Ventral ⎫	19	Intervertebral disc (between fifth and sixth cervical
4	Articular pillar	12	Dorsal ⎭ ramus		vertebra)
5	Lamina	13	Airway at level of vocal cord	20	Uncinate process
6	Spinous process of fourth cervical vertebra	14	Thyroid cartilage	21	Intervertebral foramen
7	Anterior ⎫	15	Multifidus muscle	22	Cricoid cartilage
8	Posterior ⎭ tubercle	16	Semispinalis cervicis muscle	23	Vocal cord

A and **B** Cervical spine. Axial MR images (T$_{2*}$-weighted)

1 Nucleus pulposus of intervertebral disc
2 Cerebrospinal fluid in subarachnoid space
3 White matter } of cervical spinal cord
4 Grey matter
5 Intervertebral foramen
6 Vertebral artery in transverse foramen
7 Superior articular process (facet)
8 Zygapophysial (facet joint)
9 Inferior articular process (facet)
10 Lamina
11 Multifidus muscle
12 Trachea
13 Thyroid gland
14 Common carotid artery
15 Internal jugular vein
16 Body of vertebra
17 Oesophagus
18 Longus cervicis muscle
19 Anterior longitudinal muscle and cortical bone
20 Posterior longitudinal ligament and cortical bone
21 Dorsal } ramus
22 Ventral
23 Dorsal root ganglion
24 Epidural fat
25 Spinous process
26 Ligamentum flavum
27 Sternocleidomastoid muscle
28 Trapezius muscle
29 Splenius capitis muscle
30 Semispinalis capitis muscle
31 Levator scapulae muscle

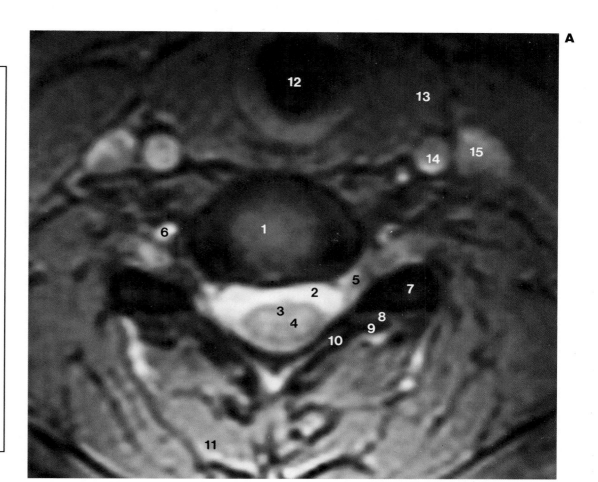

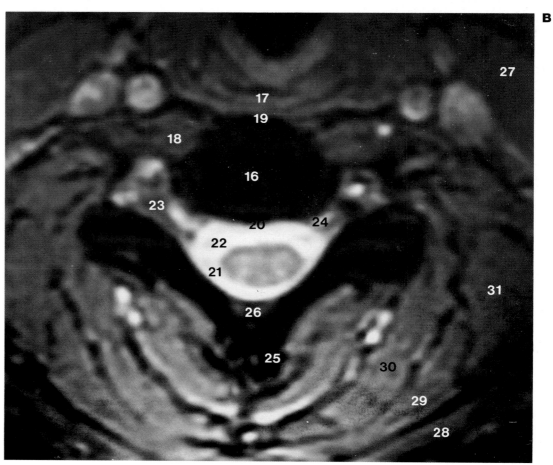

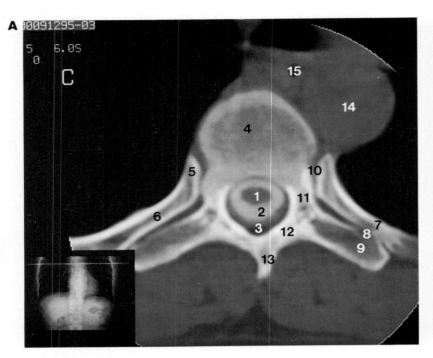

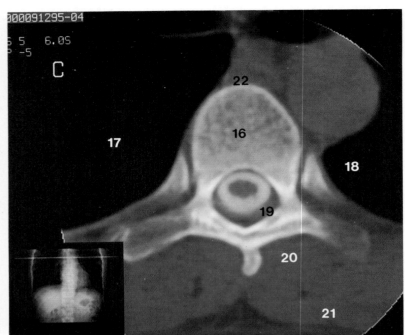

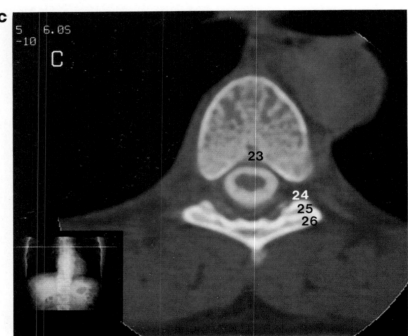

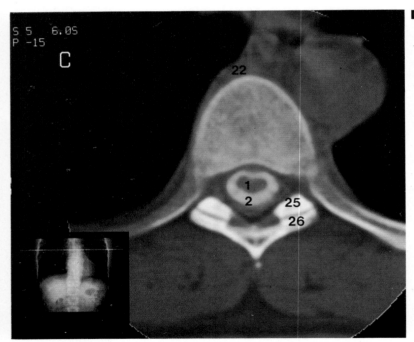

A—D Thoracic spine. Axial CT images at the level of the sixth thoracic vertebra (with intrathecal contrast medium)

1	Spinal cord	10	Costovertebral joint	20	Erector spinae muscles
2	Contrast medium in subarachnoid space	11	Pedicle	21	Trapezius muscle
3	Epidural space	12	Lamina	22	Anterior longitudinal ligament
4	Intervertebral disc (between fifth and sixth thoracic vertebrae)	13	Spinous process	23	Basivertebral veins
		14	Aorta	24	Intervertebral foramen
5	Head ⎱	15	Oesophagus	25	Superior articular process (facet) of seventh ⎱ thoracic vertebra
6	Neck ⎰ of rib	16	Body of sixth thoracic vertebra		
7	Tubercle ⎰	17	Right ⎱ lung	26	Inferior articular process (facet) of sixth ⎰
8	Costotransverse joint	18	Left ⎰		
9	Transverse process	19	Ligamentum flavum		

A Cervical spine. Sagittal MR image (T₁-weighted)

1	Spinal cord	12	Brainstem
2	Cerebrospinal fluid in subarachnoid space	13	Cervical expansion
3	Odontoid process (dens)	14	Suboccipital fat
4	Synchondrosis	15	Occipital bone
5	Body of axis (second cervical vertebra)	16	Posterior longitudinal ligament
6	Anterior ⎫ arch of atlas	17	Body of seventh cervical vertebra
7	Posterior ⎬ (first cervical vertebra)	18	Nucleus pulposus of intervertebral disc (between seventh cervical and first thoracic vertebrae)
8	Spinous process of axis		
9	Clivus	19	Anterior longitudinal ligament and cortical bone
10	Posterior margin of foramen magnum	20	Trachea
11	Cerebellar tonsil	21	Oesophagus

Thoracic spine, **B** midsagittal MR image (T₁-weighted), **C** sagittal MR image at level of intervertebral foramen (T₁-weighted), **D** sagittal MR image (T₂*-weighted)

1	Body of seventh thoracic vertebra	11	Basivertebral vein
2	Nucleus pulposus of intervertebral disc (between seventh and eighth thoracic vertebrae)	12	Posterior longitudinal ligament and annulus fibrosus
3	Spinal cord	13	Seventh thoracic nerve in intervertebral foramen
4	Cerebrospinal fluid	14	Fat in intervertebral foramen
5	Epidural fat	15	Pedicle
6	Ligamentum flavum	16	Inferior articular process of eleventh ⎫ thoracic
7	Spinous process	17	Superior articular process of twelfth ⎬ vertebra
8	Trachea	18	Facet joint
9	Anterior ⎫ longitudinal ligament and cortical bone	19	Heart
10	Posterior ⎬		

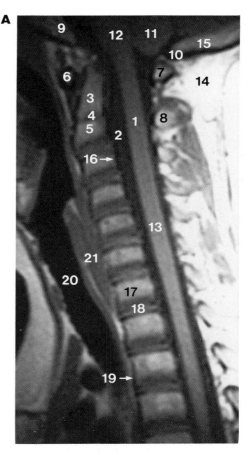

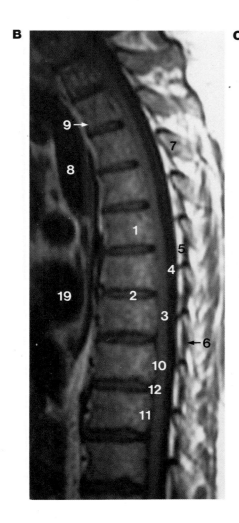

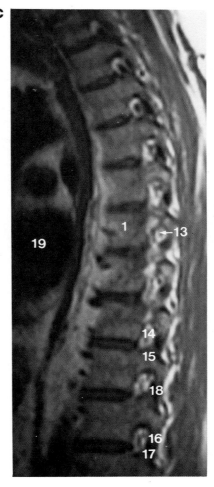

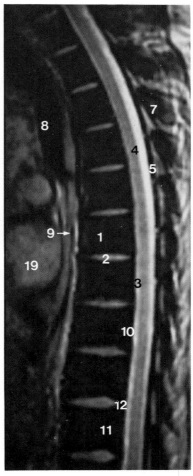

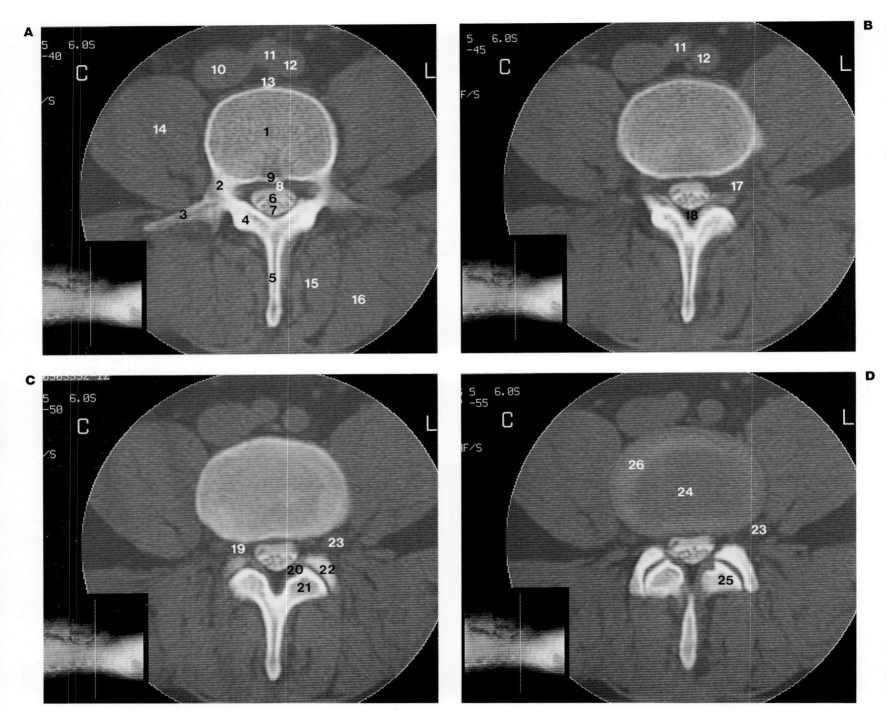

A–D Lumbar spine. Axial CT images at the level of the fourth and fifth lumbar vertebrae (with intrathecal contrast medium)
Multiple thin (5 mm) sections are taken parallel to the disc space. Lumbar epidural fat provides contrast around the theca and exiting nerve roots, and the posterior aspect of the disc.

1	Body of third lumbar vertebra	9	Basivertebral veins	18	Epidural fat
2	Pedicle	10	Inferior vena cava	19	Intervertebral foramen (between fourth and fifth lumbar vertebrae)
3	Transverse process	11	Right ⎫ common iliac artery	20	Ligamentum flavum
4	Lamina	12	Left ⎬	21	Inferior articular process (facet) of fourth ⎫ lumbar vertebra
5	Spinous process of fourth lumbar vertebra	13	Anterior longitudinal ligament	22	Superior articular process (facet) of fifth ⎬
6	Thecal sac	14	Psoas muscle	23	Root of fourth lumbar nerve
7	Nerve roots of cauda equina	15	Multifidus muscle	24	Nucleus pulposus of intervertebral disc
8	Posterior longitudinal ligament	16	Erector spinae muscle	25	Pars interarticularis
		17	Dorsal root ganglion of fourth lumbar nerve	26	Annulus fibrosus of intervertebral disc

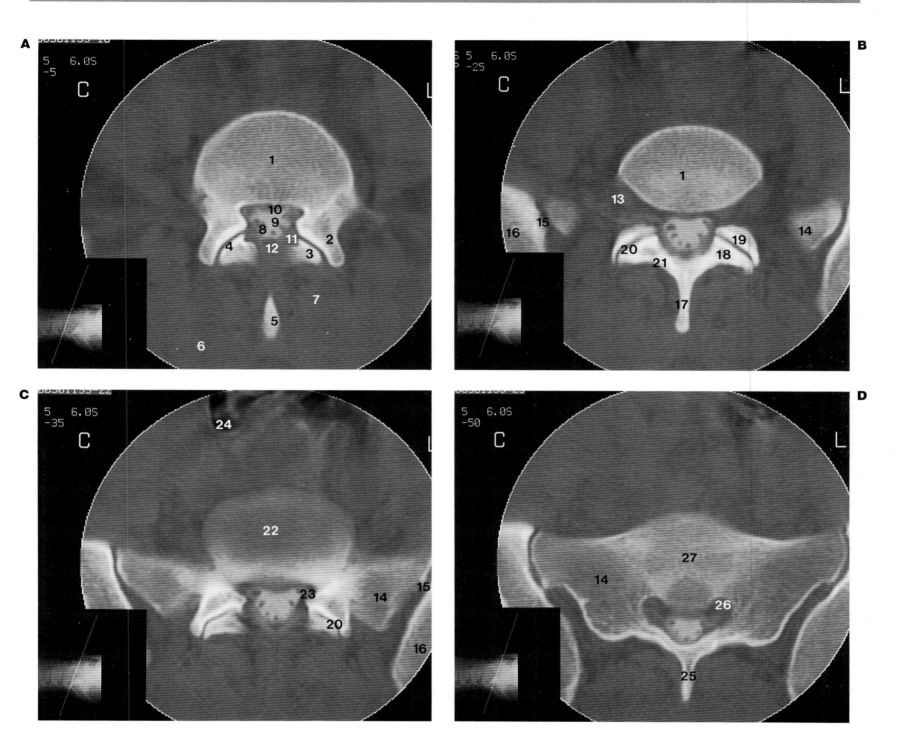

A–D Lumbar spine. Axial CT images at the level of the lumbosacral junction (with intrathecal contrast medium)

1 Body ⎱ of fifth lumbar vertebra	10 Internal vertebral veins	20 Pars interarticularis (fifth lumbar/first sacral vertebra)
2 Superior articular process (facet) ⎰	11 Ligamentum flavum	
3 Inferior articular process (facet) of fourth lumbar vertebra	12 Epidural fat	21 Lamina
4 Pars interarticularis (between fourth and fifth lumbar vertebrae)	13 Root of fifth lumbar nerve	22 Intervertebral disc (fifth lumbar/first sacral vertebra)
	14 Lateral part (ala) of sacrum	
5 Spinous process of fourth lumbar vertebra	15 Sacro-iliac joint	23 Root of first sacral nerve
6 Erector spinae muscle	16 Ilium	24 Bowel gas
7 Multifidus muscle	17 Spinous process of fifth lumbar vertebra	25 Spinous process of first sacral vertebra
8 Nerve roots of cauda equina	18 Inferior articular process (facet) of fifth lumbar vertebra	26 Sacral foramina
9 Thecal sac	19 Superior articular process (facet) of first sacral vertebra	27 Body of sacrum

A

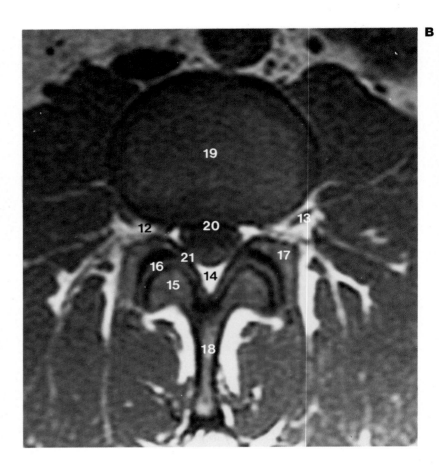

B

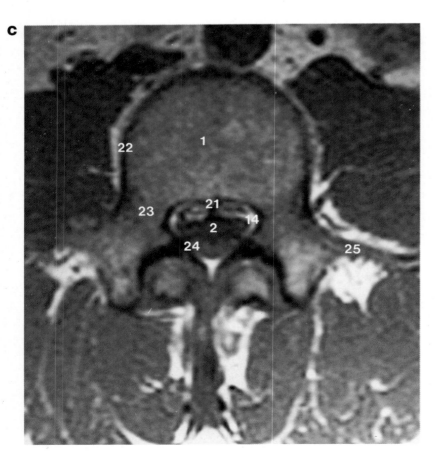

C

Lumbar spine. Axial MR images (T₁-weighted), A at the level of the body of the third lumbar vertebra, B at the level of the intervertebral disc, C at the level of the pedicles

1	Body of third lumbar vertebra
2	Cauda equina in lumbar thecal sac
3	Psoas muscle
4	Multifidus muscle
5	Inferior vena cava
6	Aorta
7	Anterior longitudinal ligament and cortical bone
8	Posterior longitudinal ligament
9	Retroperitoneal fat
10	Lamina
11	Dura
12	Fat in intervertebral foramen
13	Spinal nerve root
14	Epidural fat in epidural space
15	Inferior articular process (facet)
16	Zygapophysial (facet) joint
17	Superior articular process (facet)
18	Spinous process
19	Intervertebral disc
20	Annulus fibrosus and posterior longitudinal ligament
21	Epidural veins in epidural space
22	Cortical bone
23	Pedicle
24	Ligamentum flavum
25	Transverse process

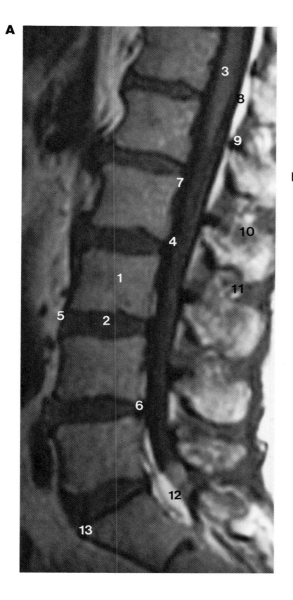

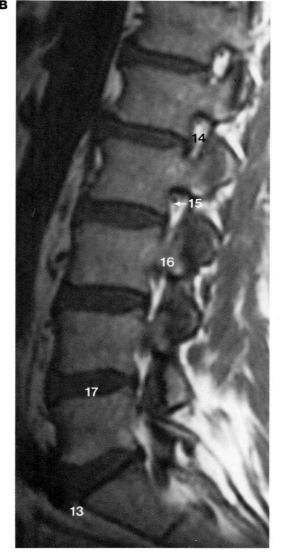

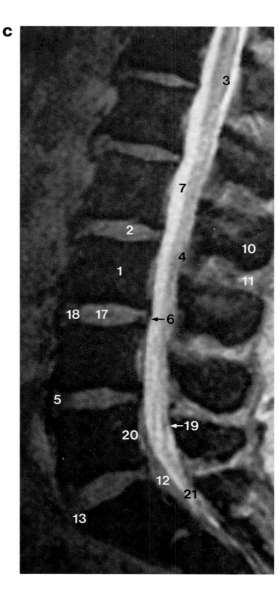

Lumbosacral spine, A midsagittal MR image (T_1-weighted), **B** sagittal MR image at level of intervertebral foramen (T_1-weighted), **C** midsagittal MR image (T_{2*}-weighted)

1	Body of third lumbar vertebra	12	Epidural space (fat filled)
2	Nucleus pulposus	13	Sacral promontory
3	Conus medullaris	14	Intervertebral foramen
4	Cauda equina	15	Spinal nerve root in intervertebral foramen
5	Anterior longitudinal ligament	16	Pedicle
6	Posterior longitudinal ligament and annulus fibrosus	17	Internuclear cleft
7	Cerebrospinal fluid	18	Annulus fibrosus
8	Epidural fat	19	Nerve root
9	Ligamentum flavum	20	Basivertebral veins
10	Spinous process	21	Caudal lumbar thecal sac
11	Interspinous ligament and bursa		

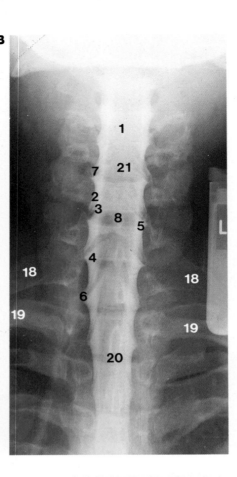

Cervical myelogram, **A** with the neck extended, **B** with the neck slightly flexed. Anteroposterior projections

Non-ionic water-soluble contrast medium is introduced into the lumbar subarachnoid space via a lumbar puncture. The patient is positioned prone, with the neck hyperextended, and strapped onto a tilting table. The contrast medium is then run up into the cervical region to demonstrate the cervical spinal cord and exiting nerve roots. There are eight cervical nerve roots: the roots of the eighth cervical nerve exit through the intervertebral foramina between the seventh cervical vertebra and the first thoracic vertebra. The normal cervical cord enlargement (8) (for the brachial plexus) extends from the third cervical vertebra to the second thoracic vertebra. It is maximal at the fifth cervical vertebra and should not be mistaken for an intramedullary lesion.

1	Cervical cord
2	Dorsal ⎫ root of spinal nerve
3	Ventral ⎭
4	Lateral margin of spinal cord
5	Contrast medium in cervical subarachnoid space
6	Root of eighth cervical nerve
7	Cervical spinal nerve exiting through intervertebral foramen
8	Cervical cord enlargement
9	Odontoid process (dens)
10	Transverse foramen
11	Lateral mass of atlas (first cervical vertebra)
12	Vertebral artery
13	Basilar artery
14	Posterior inferior cerebellar artery
15	Radicular artery
16	Mandible
17	Occiput
18	Normal large transverse process of seventh cervical vertebra
19	First rib
20	Thoracic cord
21	Anterior spinal artery

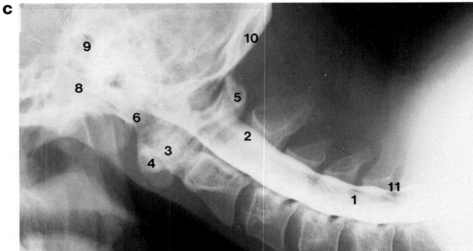

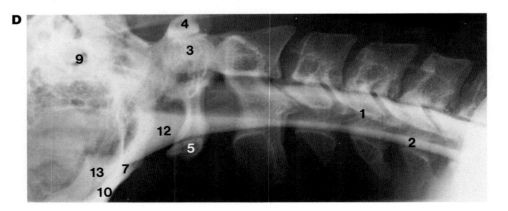

Cervical myelogram, **C** with the patient prone, **D** with the patient supine. Lateral projections

1	Cervical cord
2	Contrast medium in cervical subarachnoid space
3	Odontoid (process) dens
4	Anterior arch ⎫ of atlas (first cervical vertebra)
5	Posterior tubercle ⎭
6	Anterior ⎫ rim of foramen magnum
7	Posterior ⎭
8	Clivus
9	External acoustic meatus
10	Occiput
11	Posterior indentation on theca from ligamentum flavum
12	Posterior inferior cerebellar artery
13	Cisterna magna (cerebellomedullary cistern)

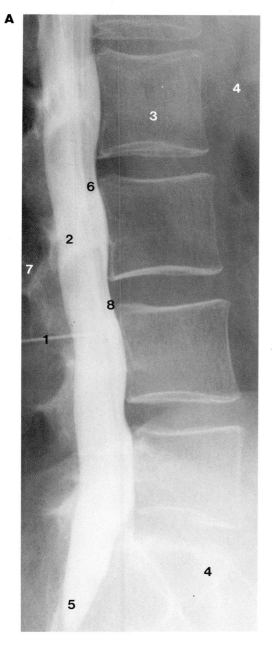

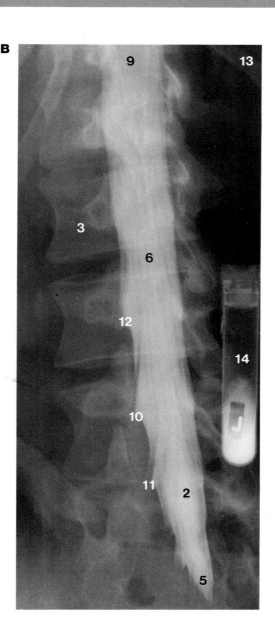

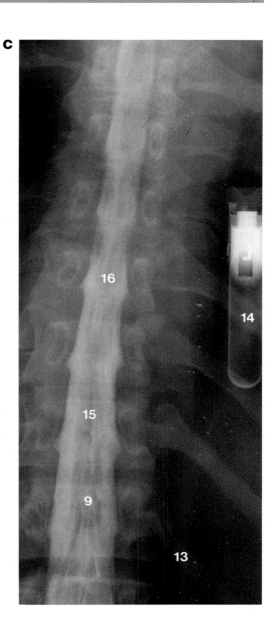

Lumbar radiculogram, A lateral projection, B oblique projection, C anteroposterior projection

Non-ionic water-soluble contrast medium is introduced into the lumbar subarachnoid space via a lumbar puncture. The nerve roots of the cauda equina are well demonstrated and exit through the intervertebral foramina. The nerve roots extending from the conus to the terminal thecal sac pass below the pedicle of the corresponding vertebra. The thecal sac terminates at the level of the first/second sacral vertebra. The filum terminale may be seen. Tilting the prone patient slightly head down allows the contrast to flow cranially and outlines the conus and lower thoracic cord. The cord is uniform in size from the second to the tenth thoracic vertebra, at which point its second, smaller expansion (for the lumbosacral plexus) extends from the tenth thoracic vertebra to the level of the first lumbar vertebra. The conus medullaris usually terminates at the first/second lumbar vertebra, but may be seen at a level above and below as a normal variant.

1	Lumbar puncture needle in space between third and fourth lumbar vertebrae
2	Contrast medium in subarachnoid space
3	Body of second lumbar vertebra
4	Sacral promontory
5	Terminal theca at first/second sacral vertebra
6	Spinal nerves within subarachnoid space (cauda equina)
7	Spinous process of third lumbar vertebra
8	Intervertebral disc indentations on anterior thecal margin
9	Conus medullaris
10	Fourth ⎱ lumbar spinal nerve
11	Fifth ⎰
12	Lateral extension of subarachnoid space around spinal nerve roots
13	Twelfth rib
14	Test tube containing contrast medium to indicate tilt of patient
15	Anterior median fissure
16	Thoracic cord

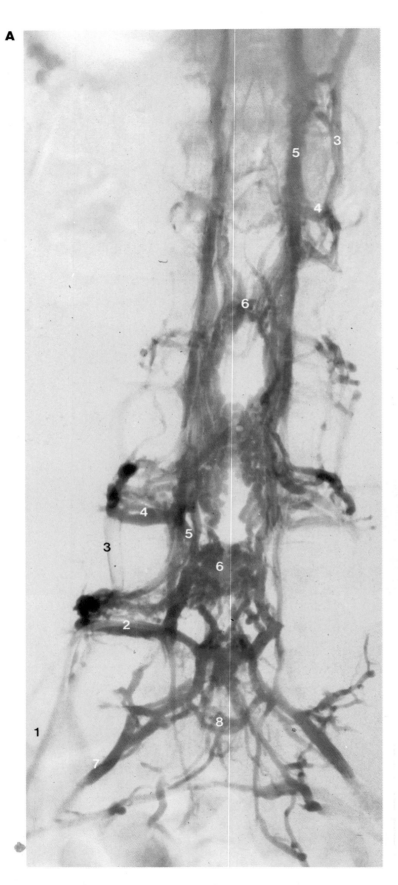

A Subtracted lumbar venogram

Since the advent of CT and MR imaging techniques, lumbar venography is rarely performed. However, the anatomy of the vertebral veins is optimally demonstrated by this technique. Venous drainage of the spinal cord is longitudinally arranged via plexi, which anastomose freely with the internal (5) and external (3 and 4) vertebral venous plexi, which also communicate (4 and 6). Note how the internal veins bend laterally at the level of the disc interspace and medially at the level of pedicles, where they unite via a connecting vein (6).

1	Catheter in common iliac vein
2	Tip of catheter in intravertebral vein
3	Ascending lumbar veins
4	Intervertebral veins
5	Longitudinal vertebral venous plexi
6	Basivertebral veins
7	Lateral sacral vein
8	Sacral venous plexus

B Spinal arteriogram

1	Selective catheterisation of left eleventh intercostal artery
2	Arteria radicularis magna (Adamkiewicz)
3	Anterior spinal artery
4	Normal transdural stenosis of the arteria radicularis magna

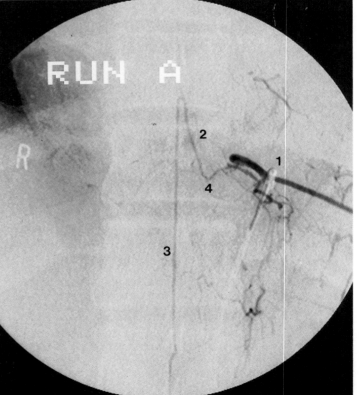

Upper limb

A Shoulder. Anteroposterior radiograph

1	Clavicle	
2	Scapula	
3	Glenoid fossa	
4	Coracoid process	of scapula
5	Acromion	
6	Head	
7	Greater tubercle (tuberosity)	
8	Intertubercular groove	of humerus
9	Lesser tubercle (tuberosity)	
10	Anatomical neck	
11	Surgical neck	

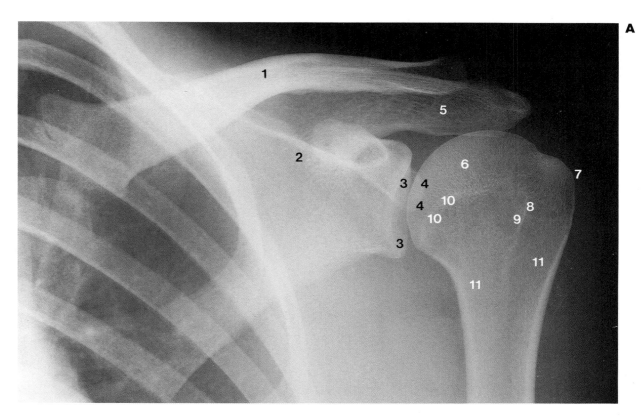

B Shoulder. Axial (supero-inferior) projection

1	Clavicle	
2	Spine	
3	Coracoid process	of scapula
4	Glenoid fossa	
5	Acromion	
6	Head	
7	Lesser tubercle (tuberosity)	
8	Intertubercular groove	of humerus
9	Greater tubercle (tuberosity)	

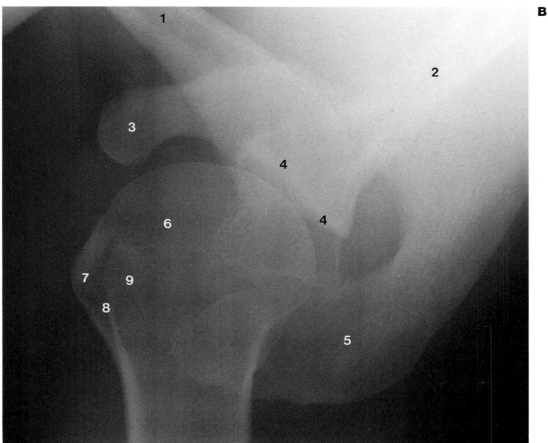

69

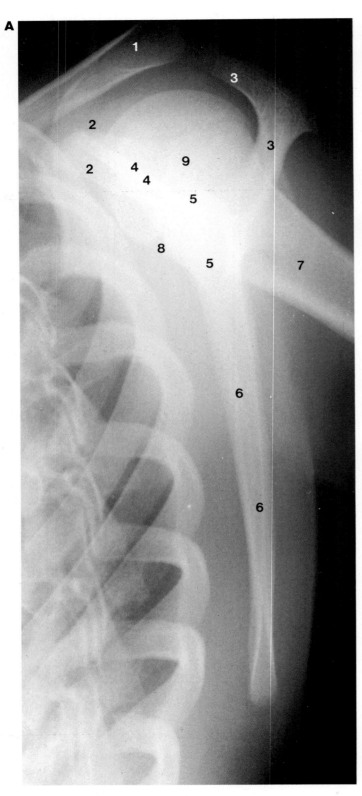

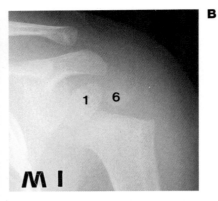

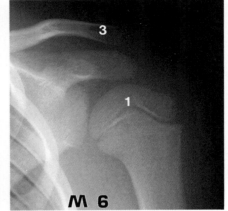

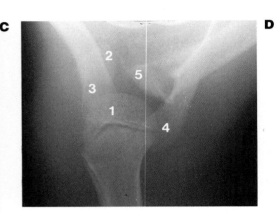

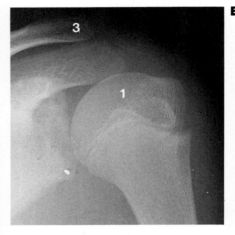

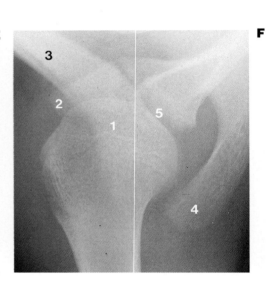

Shoulder, **B** (anteroposterior) of a
1-year-old child, **C** (anteroposterior)
and **D** (axial) of a 6-year-old child,
E (anteroposterior) and **F** (axial) of
a 14-year-old child

1	Centre for head of humerus
2	Centre for coracoid process
3	Clavicle
4	Acromion
5	Glenoid fossa
6	Centre for greater tubercle (tuberosity) of humerus

A Scapula of a 14-year-old boy. Lateral projection

1	Clavicle	6	Lateral border of scapula
2	Coracoid process	7	Humerus
3	Acromion	8	Epiphysial line
4	Spine of scapula	9	Head of humerus
5	Glenoid fossa		

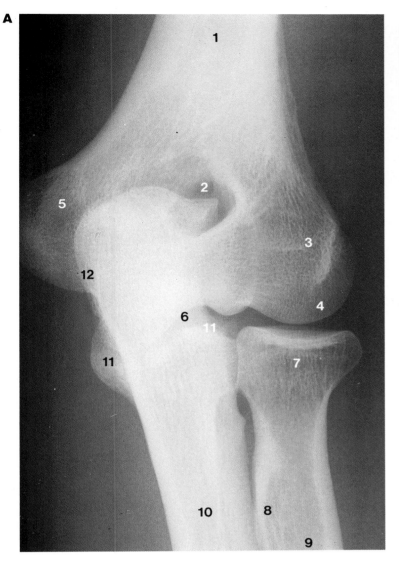

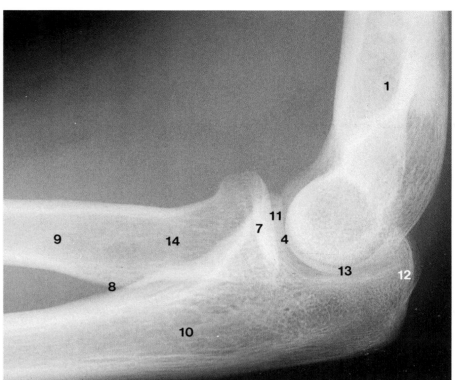

Elbow, A anteroposterior projection, **B** lateral projection, **C** axial projection

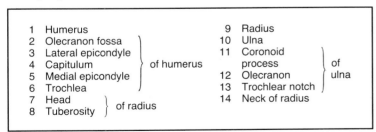

1	Humerus		9	Radius	
2	Olecranon fossa		10	Ulna	
3	Lateral epicondyle		11	Coronoid	
4	Capitulum	of humerus		process	of
5	Medial epicondyle		12	Olecranon	ulna
6	Trochlea		13	Trochlear notch	
7	Head	of radius	14	Neck of radius	
8	Tuberosity				

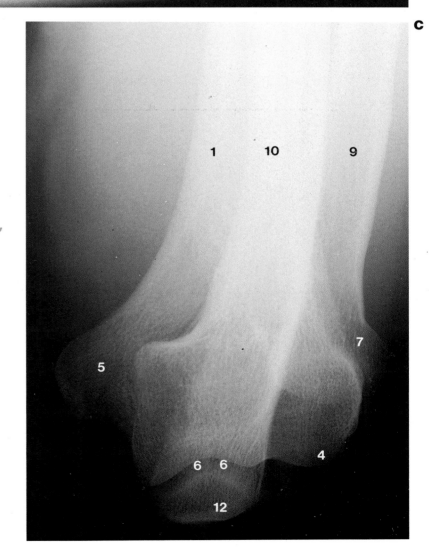

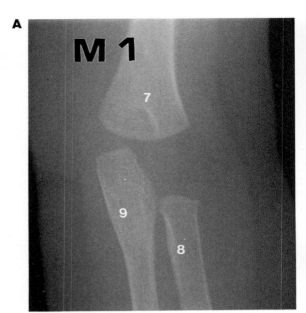

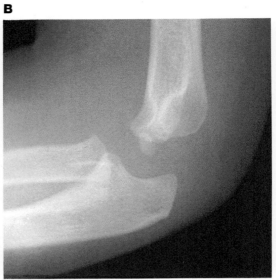

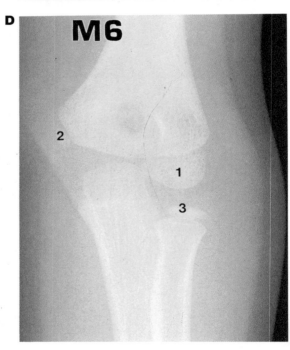

Elbow, **A** (anteroposterior) of a 1-year-old child, **B** (lateral) and **C** (anteroposterior) of a 3-year-old child, **D** (anteroposterior) of a 6-year-old child, **E** (anteroposterior) of a 9-year-old child, **F** (lateral) of 11-year-old child, **G** (lateral) and **H** (anteroposterior) of a 14-year-old child, to illustrate centres of ossification

1	Centre for capitulum
2	Centre for medial epicondyle
3	Centre for radial head
4	Centre for trochlea
5	Centre for olecranon
6	Centre for lateral epicondyle
7	Humerus
8	Radius
9	Ulna

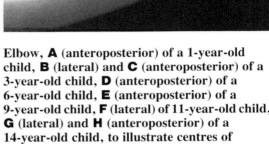

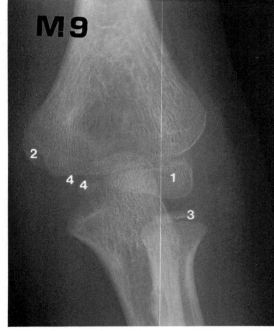

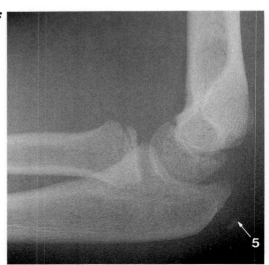

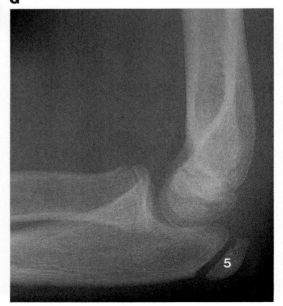

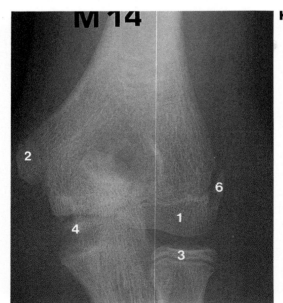

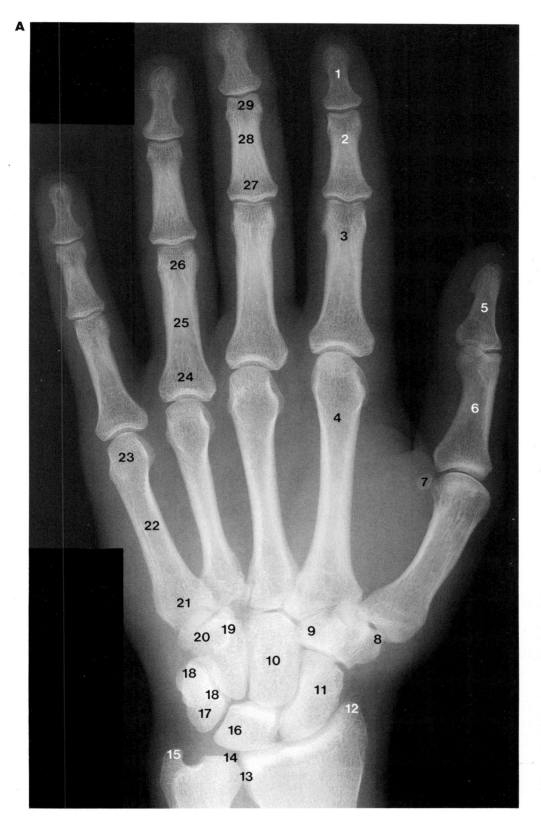

A Bones of the hand. Dorsopalmar projection

1	Distal	⎫
2	Middle	⎬ phalanx of index finger
3	Proximal	⎭
4	Second metacarpal	
5	Distal	⎫ phalanx
6	Proximal	⎬ of thumb
7	Sesamoid bone	
8	Trapezium	
9	Trapezoid	
10	Capitate	
11	Scaphoid	
12	Styloid process	⎫ of radius
13	Ulnar notch	⎬
14	Head	⎫ of ulna
15	Styloid process	⎬
16	Lunate	
17	Triquetral	
18	Pisiform	
19	Hook of hamate	
20	Hamate	
21	Base	⎫
22	Shaft	⎬ of fifth metacarpal
23	Head	⎭
24	Base	⎫ of proximal phalanx
25	Shaft	⎬ of ring finger
26	Head	⎭
27	Base	⎫ of middle phalanx
28	Shaft	⎬ of middle finger
29	Head	⎭
30	Radius	

● There are often two sesamoids (7), present in the flexor pollicis brevis and adductor pollicis muscles.

B Bones of the wrist. Lateral projection

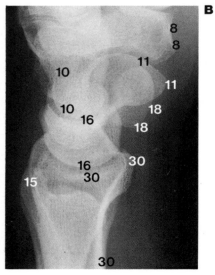

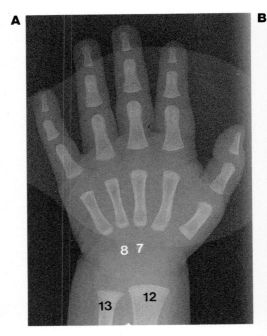

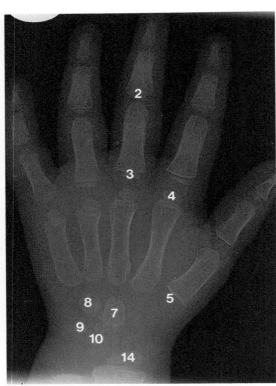

Bones of the hand (dorsopalmar projections), A of a 3-month-old boy, **B** of a 3-year-old boy, **C** of a 6-year-old boy, **D** of an 11-year-old boy, to illustrate centres of ossification

1	Centre for distal ⎫
2	Centre for middle ⎬ phalanx of middle finger
3	Centre for proximal ⎭
4	Centre for second metacarpal (applies to second to fifth metacarpals)
5	Centre for first metacarpal
6	Trapezium
7	Capitate
8	Hamate
9	Triquetral
10	Lunate
11	Scaphoid
12	Radius
13	Ulna
14	Centre for distal radius
15	Trapezoid
16	Centre for distal ulna

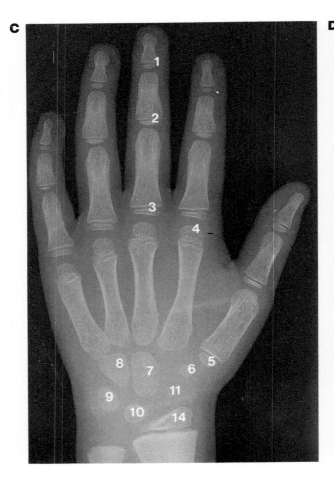

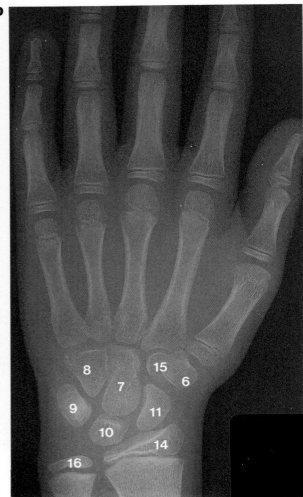

Axillary arteriograms. A subtracted, B digitally subtracted

1　Axillary artery
2　Superior thoracic artery
3　Lateral thoracic artery
4　Subscapular artery
5　Posterior circumflex humeral artery
6　Anterior circumflex humeral artery
7　Brachial artery
8　Muscular branches of brachial artery
9　Profunda brachii artery
10　Thoraco-acromial artery

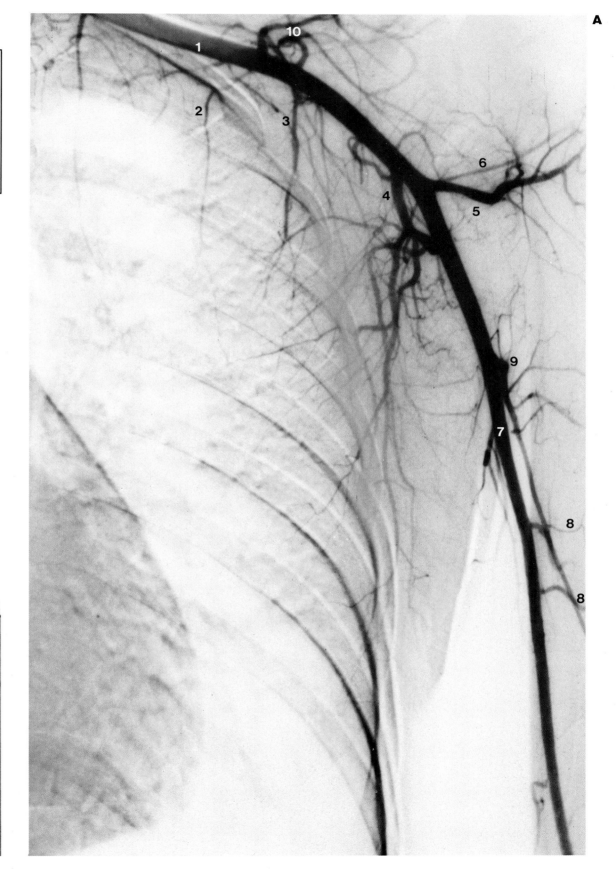

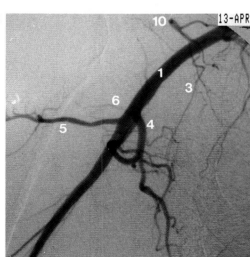

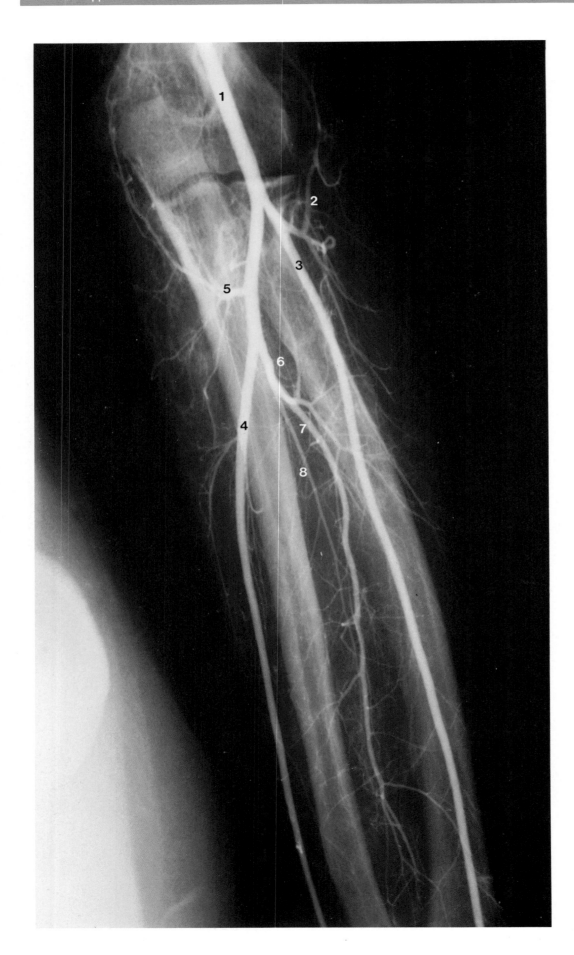

Brachial arteriogram

1 Brachial artery
2 Radial recurrent artery
3 Radial artery
4 Ulnar artery
5 Ulnar recurrent artery
6 Common interosseous artery
7 Anterior interosseous artery
8 Posterior interosseous artery

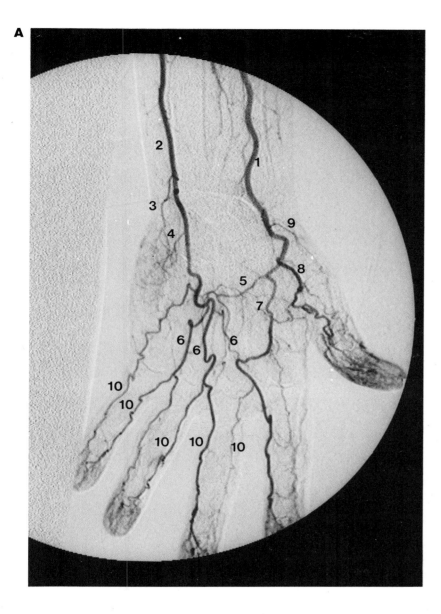

A Digitally subtracted hand arteriogram

In this patient there is an incomplete superficial palmar arch

1	Radial artery
2	Ulnar artery
3	Deep palmar branch of ulnar artery
4	Palmar carpal branch of ulnar artery
5	Deep palmar arch
6	Common palmar digital arteries
7	Palmar metacarpal artery
8	Princeps pollicis artery
9	Artery to radial aspect of thumb
10	Proper palmar digital artery

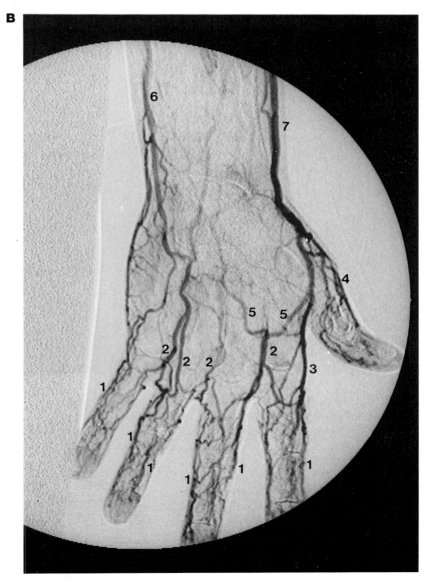

B Venous phase of hand arteriogram

1	Palmar digital veins
2	Common palmar digital veins
3	Radialis indicis vein
4	Princeps pollicis vein
5	Superficial palmar venous arch
6	Basilic vein
7	Cephalic vein

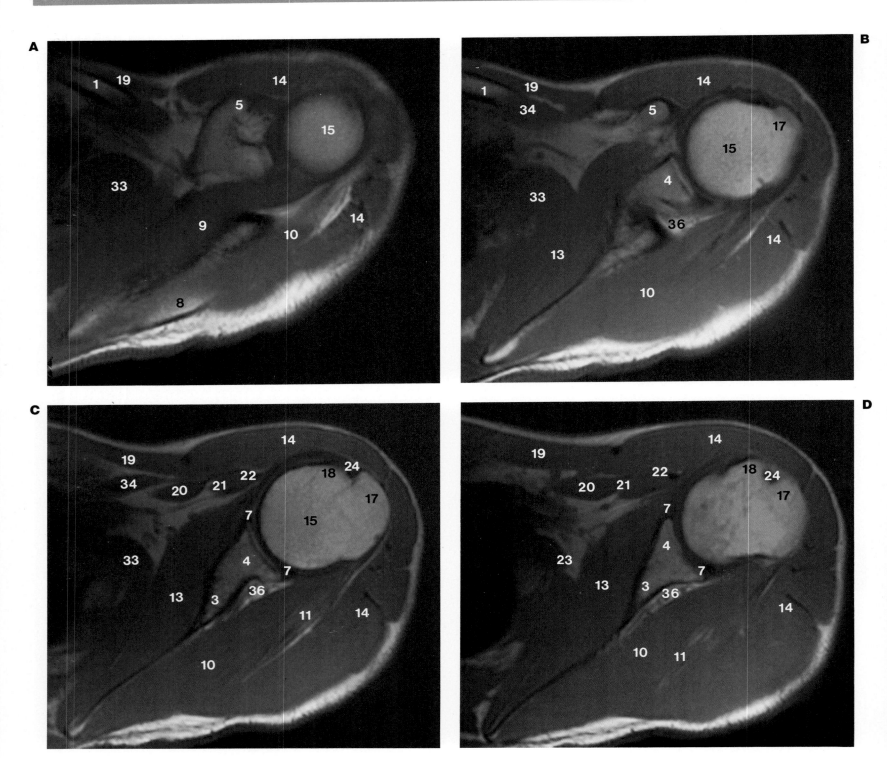

A–L Shoulder. MR images
A–F Axial images (T$_1$-weighted)
G and **H** Oblique sagittal images (T$_1$-weighted)

1	Clavicle	7	Glenoid labrum	13	Subscapularis muscle
2	Acromion	8	Spine of scapula	14	Deltoid muscle
3	Body of scapula	9	Supraspinatus muscle	15	Head } of humerus
4	Glenoid fossa	10	Infraspinatus muscle	16	Shaft } of humerus
5	Coracoid process	11	Teres minor muscle	17	Greater } tuberosity
6	Acromioclavicular joint	12	Teres major muscle	18	Lesser } tuberosity

E 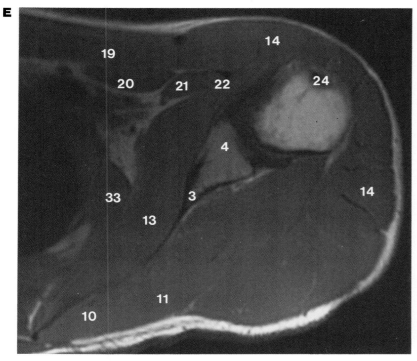 F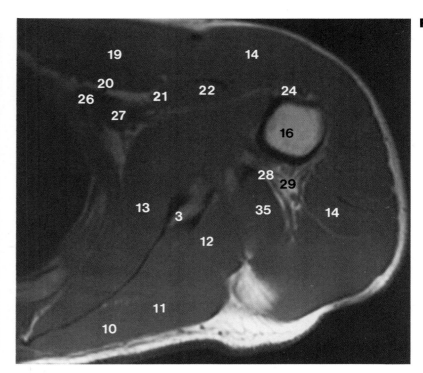

G 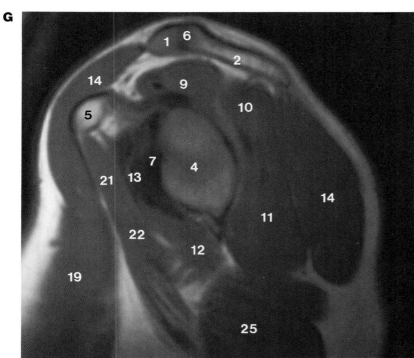 H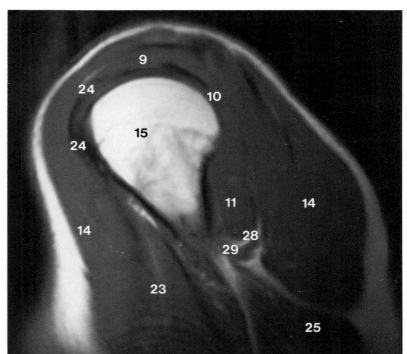

19	Pectoralis major muscle	25	Latissimus dorsi muscle	31	Coracoclavicular ligament (trapezoid)
20	Pectoralis minor muscle	26	Axillary artery and vein	32	Tendon of supraspinatus muscle
21	Coracobrachialis muscle	27	Cords of brachial plexus	33	Serratus anterior muscle
22	Short head	28	Posterior circumflex humeral artery	34	Subclavius muscle
23	Long head } of biceps brachii muscle	29	Axillary nerve	35	Long head of triceps muscle
24	Tendon of long head	30	Trapezius muscle	36	Suprascapular artery

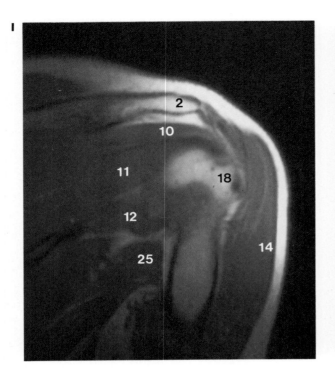

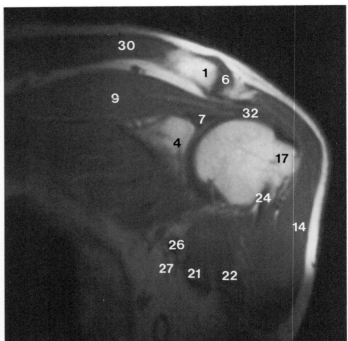

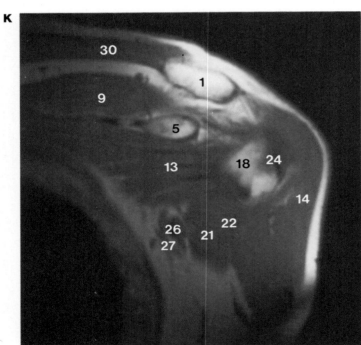

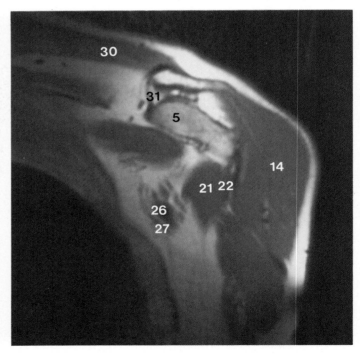

I—L Oblique coronal images (T$_1$-weighted)

1	Clavicle	10	Infraspinatus muscle	19	Pectoralis major muscle	28	Posterior circumflex humeral artery
2	Acromion	11	Teres minor muscle	20	Pectoralis minor muscle	29	Axillary nerve
3	Body of scapula	12	Teres major muscle	21	Coracobrachialis muscle	30	Trapezius muscle
4	Glenoid fossa	13	Subscapularis muscle	22	Short head	of biceps brachii muscle	31	Coracoclavicular ligament (trapezoid)
5	Coracoid process	14	Deltoid muscle	23	Long head	32	Tendon of supraspinatus muscle
6	Acromioclavicular joint	15	Head	of humerus	24	Tendon of long head	33	Serratus anterior muscle
7	Glenoid labrum	16	Shaft	25	Latissimus dorsi muscle	34	Subclavius muscle
8	Spine of scapula	17	Greater	tuberosity	26	Axillary artery and vein	35	Long head of triceps muscle
9	Supraspinatus muscle	18	Lesser	27	Cords of brachial plexus	36	Suprascapular artery

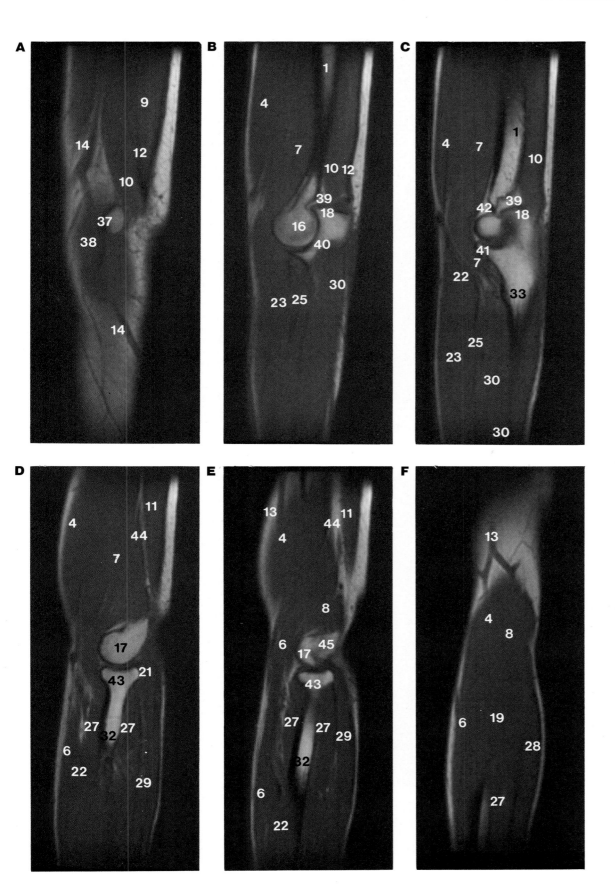

1	Humerus
2	Lateral ⎱ supracondylar ridge
3	Medial ⎰
4	Biceps brachii muscle
5	Tendon of biceps brachii muscle
6	Brachioradialis muscle
7	Brachialis muscle
8	Extensor carpi radialis longus muscle
9	Long head ⎱
10	Medial head ⎰ of triceps muscle
11	Lateral head ⎰
12	Tendon of triceps muscle
13	Cephalic vein
14	Basilic vein
15	Brachial artery
16	Trochlea ⎱ of humerus
17	Capitulum ⎰
18	Olecranon process of ulna
19	Extensor carpi radialis brevis muscle
20	Common extensor origin
21	Anconeus muscle
22	Pronator teres muscle
23	Flexor carpi radialis muscle
24	Palmaris longus muscle
25	Flexor digitorum superficialis muscle
26	Flexor carpi ulnaris muscle
27	Supinator muscle
28	Extensor digitorum muscle
29	Extensor carpi ulnaris muscle
30	Flexor digitorum profundus muscle
31	Ulnar nerve
32	Radius
33	Ulna
34	Radial nerve
35	Ulnar artery
36	Interosseous membrane
37	Medial epicondyle
38	Common flexor origin
39	Olecranon fossa ⎱ of humerus
40	Trochlear notch ⎰
41	Coronoid process ⎱
42	Coronoid fossa ⎰ of radius
43	Head ⎰
44	Lateral intermuscular septum
45	Lateral epicondyle
46	Tuberosity of radius
47	Radial notch

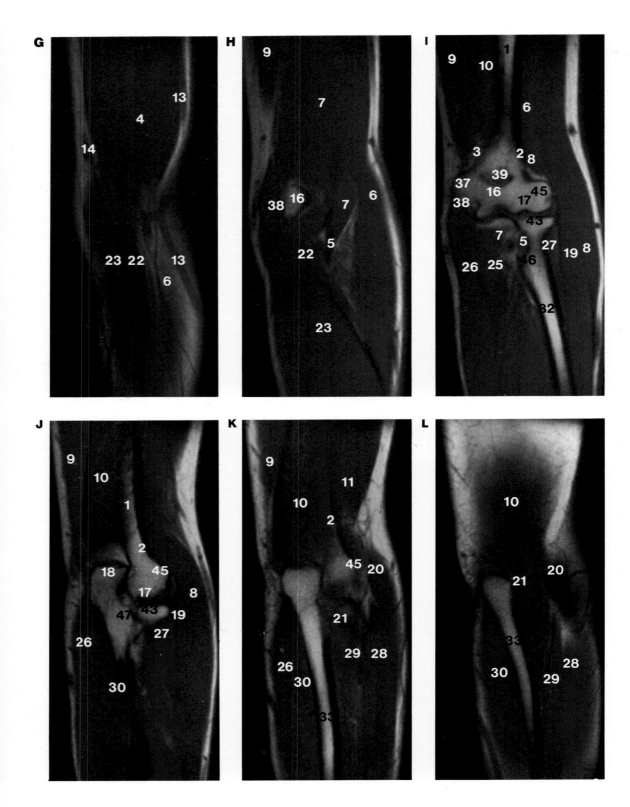

1 Humerus
2 Lateral ⎫
3 Medial ⎬ supracondylar ridge
4 Biceps brachii muscle
5 Tendon of biceps brachii muscle
6 Brachioradialis muscle
7 Brachialis muscle
8 Extensor carpi radialis longus muscle
9 Long head ⎫
10 Medial head ⎬ of triceps muscle
11 Lateral head ⎭
12 Tendon of triceps muscle
13 Cephalic vein
14 Basilic vein
15 Brachial vein
16 Trochlea ⎫
17 Capitulum ⎬ of humerus
18 Olecranon process of ulna
19 Extensor carpi radialis brevis muscle
20 Common extensor origin
21 Anconeus muscle
22 Pronator teres muscle
23 Flexor carpi radialis muscle
24 Palmaris longus muscle
25 Flexor digitorum superficialis muscle
26 Flexor carpi ulnaris muscle
27 Supinator muscle
28 Extensor digitorum muscle
29 Extensor carpi ulnaris muscle
30 Flexor digitorum profundus muscle
31 Ulnar nerve
32 Radius
33 Ulna
34 Radial nerve
35 Ulnar artery
36 Interosseous membrane
37 Medial epicondyle
38 Common flexor origin
39 Olecranon fossa ⎫
40 Trochlear notch ⎬ of humerus
41 Coronoid process ⎭
42 Coronoid fossa ⎫ of radius
43 Head ⎭
44 Lateral intermuscular septum
45 Lateral epicondyle
46 Tuberosity of radius
47 Radial notch

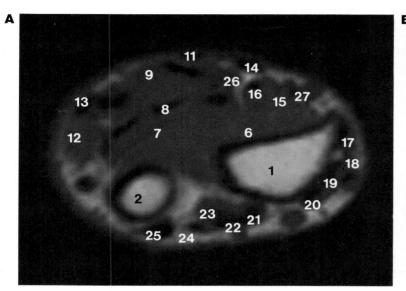

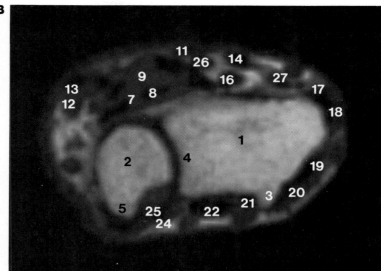

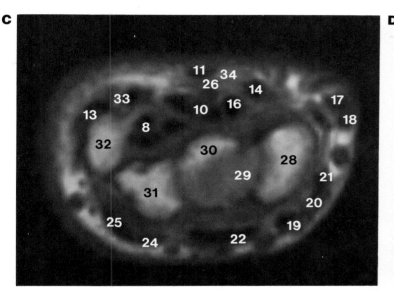

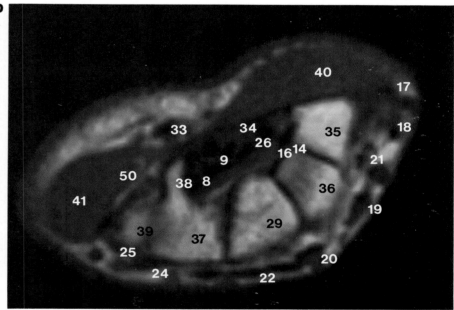

A–L Wrist and hand. MR images
A–D Axial images (T$_1$-weighted)

1	Radius	21	Tendon of extensor pollicis longus muscle	41	Abductor digiti minimi muscle
2	Ulna	22	Tendon of extensor digitorum muscle	42	Base of first
3	Dorsal tubercle } of radius	23	Tendon of extensor indicis muscle	43	Base of second
4	Ulnar notch	24	Tendon of extensor digiti minimi muscle	44	Base of third } metacarpal
5	Styloid process of ulna	25	Tendon of extensor carpi ulnaris muscle	45	Base of fourth
6	Pronator quadratus muscle	26	Median nerve	46	Metacarpal shaft
7	Flexor digitorum profundus muscle	27	Radial artery	47	Opponens pollicis muscle
8	Tendon of flexor digitorum profundus muscle	28	Scaphoid	48	Flexor pollicis brevis muscle
9	Flexor digitorum superficialis muscle	29	Capitate	49	Adductor pollicis muscle
10	Tendon of flexor digitorum superficialis muscle	30	Lunate	50	Flexor digiti minimi muscle
11	Tendon of palmaris longus muscle	31	Triquetral	51	Opponens digiti minimi muscle
12	Flexor carpi ulnaris muscle	32	Pisiform	52	Dorsal interossei muscles
13	Tendon of flexor carpi ulnaris muscle	33	Ulnar artery	53	Ventral interossei muscles
14	Tendon of flexor carpi radialis muscle	34	Flexor retinaculum	54	Lumbrical muscle
15	Flexor pollicis longus muscle	35	Trapezium	55	Superficial palmar arch
16	Tendon of flexor pollicis longus muscle	36	Trapezoid	56	Base } of proximal phalanx
17	Tendon of abductor pollicis longus muscle	37	Hamate	57	Shaft
18	Tendon of extensor pollicis brevis muscle	38	Hook of hamate	58	Middle } phalanx
19	Tendon of extensor carpi radialis longus muscle	39	Base of fifth metacarpal	59	Distal
20	Tendon of extensor carpi radialis brevis muscle	40	Abductor pollicis brevis muscle		

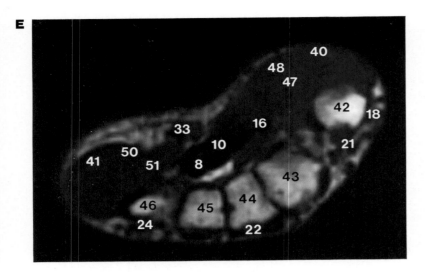

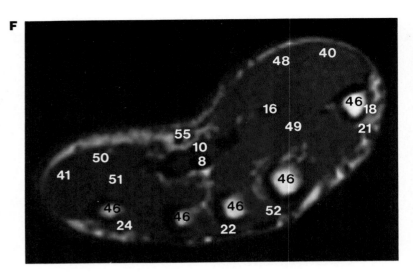

E and **F** Axial images (T$_1$-weighted)

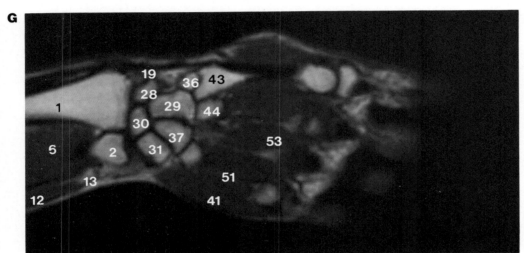

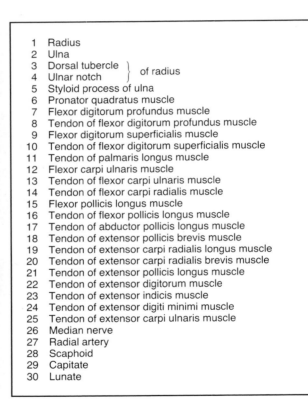

1	Radius
2	Ulna
3	Dorsal tubercle ⎫
4	Ulnar notch ⎭ of radius
5	Styloid process of ulna
6	Pronator quadratus muscle
7	Flexor digitorum profundus muscle
8	Tendon of flexor digitorum profundus muscle
9	Flexor digitorum superficialis muscle
10	Tendon of flexor digitorum superficialis muscle
11	Tendon of palmaris longus muscle
12	Flexor carpi ulnaris muscle
13	Tendon of flexor carpi ulnaris muscle
14	Tendon of flexor carpi radialis muscle
15	Flexor pollicis longus muscle
16	Tendon of flexor pollicis longus muscle
17	Tendon of abductor pollicis longus muscle
18	Tendon of extensor pollicis brevis muscle
19	Tendon of extensor carpi radialis longus muscle
20	Tendon of extensor carpi radialis brevis muscle
21	Tendon of extensor pollicis longus muscle
22	Tendon of extensor digitorum muscle
23	Tendon of extensor indicis muscle
24	Tendon of extensor digiti minimi muscle
25	Tendon of extensor carpi ulnaris muscle
26	Median nerve
27	Radial artery
28	Scaphoid
29	Capitate
30	Lunate

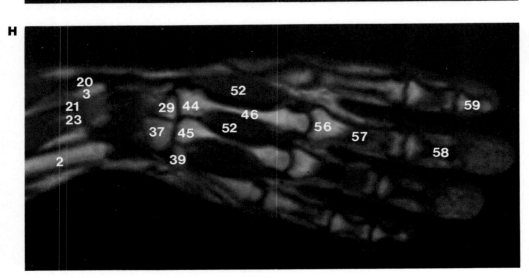

G and **H** Coronal images (T$_1$-weighted)

I—L Sagittal images (T$_1$-weighted)

31 Triquetral
32 Pisiform
33 Ulnar artery
34 Flexor retinaculum
35 Trapezium
36 Trapezoid
37 Hamate
38 Hook of hamate
39 Base of fifth metacarpal
40 Abductor pollicis brevis muscle
41 Abductor digiti minimi muscle
42 Base of first ⎫
43 Base of second ⎬ metacarpal
44 Base of third ⎪
45 Base of fourth ⎭
46 Metacarpal shaft
47 Opponens pollicis muscle
48 Flexor pollicis brevis muscle
49 Adductor pollicis muscle
50 Flexor digiti minimi muscle
51 Opponens digiti minimi muscle
52 Dorsal interossei muscles
53 Ventral interossei muscles
54 Lumbrical muscle
55 Superficial palmar arch
56 Base ⎫ of proximal phalanx
57 Shaft ⎭
58 Middle ⎫ phalanx
59 Distal ⎭

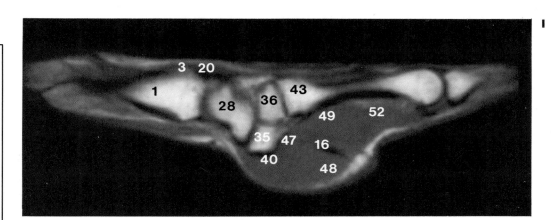
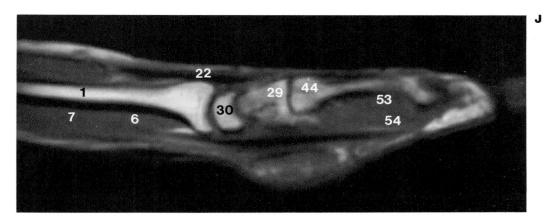
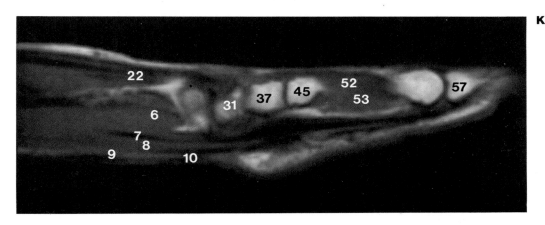
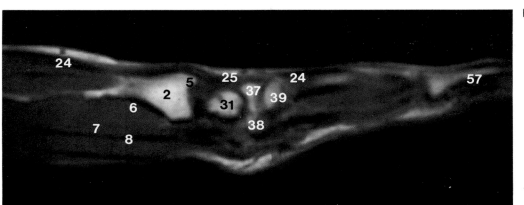

Thorax

A Chest of a 4-month-old child. Postero-anterior radiograph

1	Thymus
2	Cervical rib
3	Azygos fissure

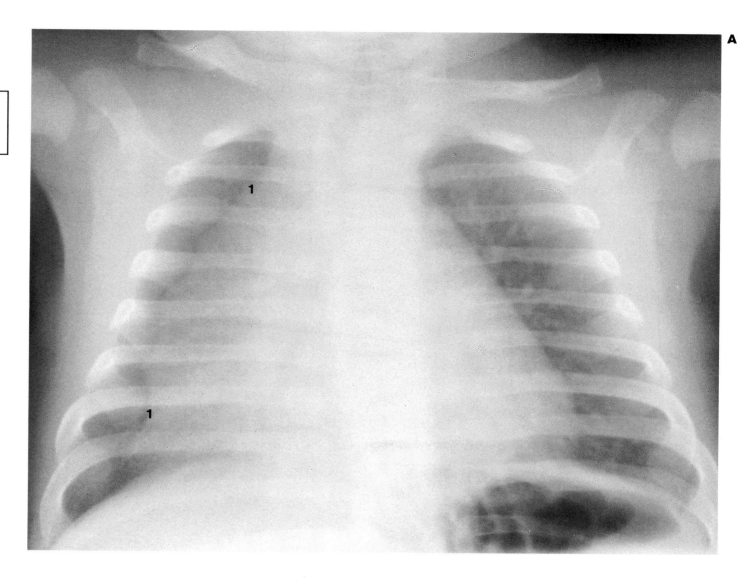

A

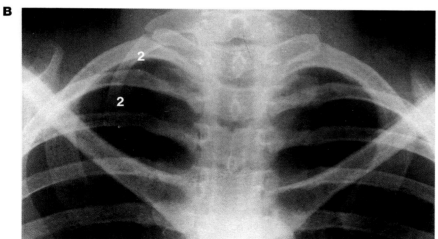

B Cervical rib. Postero-anterior projection

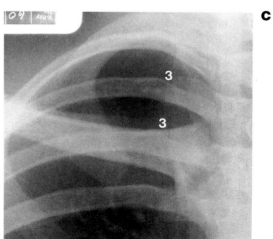

C Azygos fissure. Postero-anterior projection

87

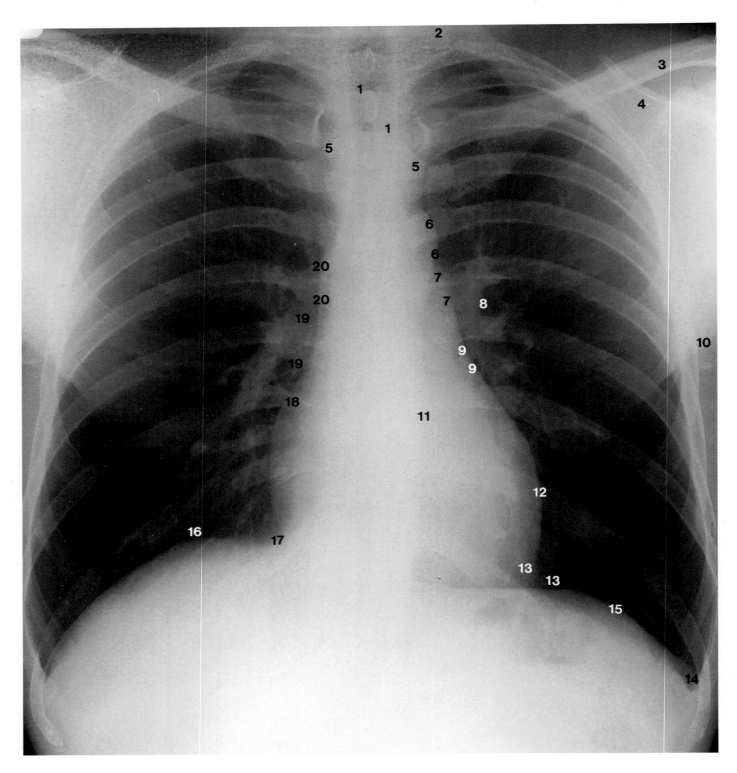

Chest of an adult male. Postero-anterior projection

1	Trachea	8	Left pulmonary artery	15	Left	dome of diaphragm
2	First rib	9	Region of tip of auricle of left atrium	16	Right	
3	Clavicle	10	Anterior axillary fold	17	Inferior vena cava	
4	Spine of scapula	11	Descending aorta	18	Right atrial border	
5	Sternum	12	Border of left ventricle	19	Right pulmonary artery	
6	Arch of aorta (aortic knuckle or knob)	13	Left cardiophrenic angle	20	Superior vena cava	
7	Pulmonary trunk	14	Left costophrenic angle			

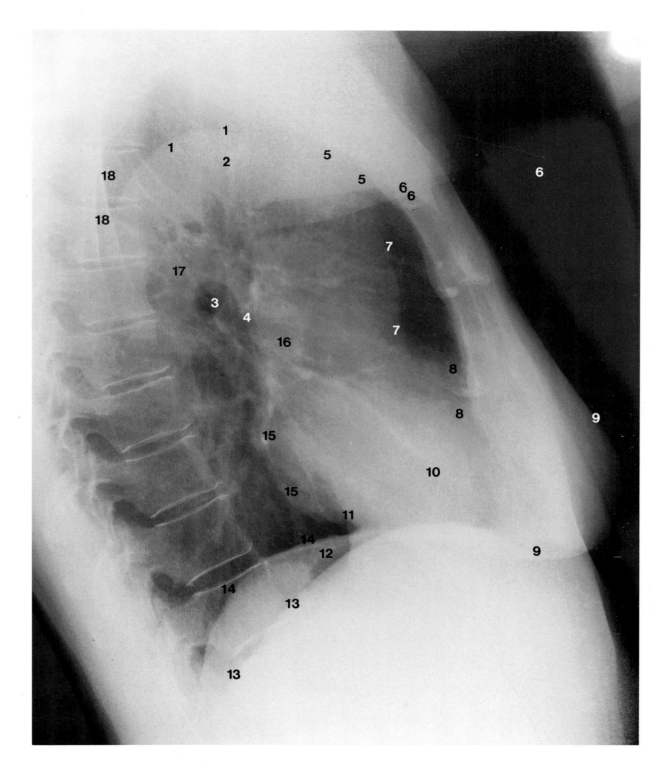

Chest of an adult female. Lateral projection

1	Arch of aorta (aortic knuckle or knob)	7	Infundibulum of right ventricle (below) with pulmonary trunk (above)	13	Right	dome of diaphragm
2	Trachea	8	Right ventricular border of heart	14	Left	
3	Left	main bronchus	9	Breast	15	Left atrial border of heart
4	Right		10	Left oblique fissure	16	Right	main pulmonary artery
5	Ascending aorta	11	Inferior vena cava	17	Left	
6	Soft tissues of upper arm	12	Gas in fundus of stomach	18	Scapula	

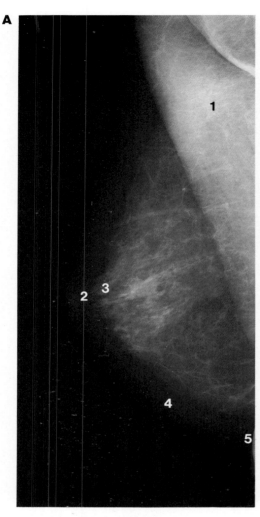

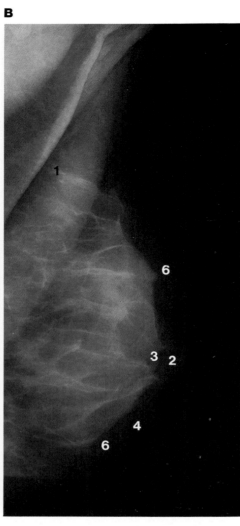

A Postmenopausal right breast. Lateral oblique mammogram

B Premenopausal left breast. Lateral oblique mammogram

1	Pectoral muscles
2	Nipple
3	Subareolar area
4	Line of skin
5	Inframammary fold
6	Suspensory ligament (Cooper's)
7	Lactiferous duct
8	Lactiferous sinus
9	Lobar duct pattern (comprising (intra) lobar ducts and terminal ductal lobular units)
10	Right ⎫
11	Left ⎭ breast

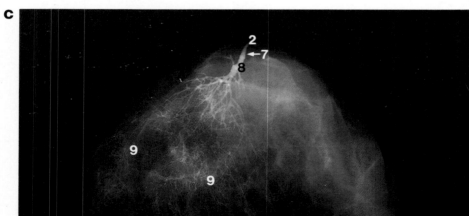

C Premenopausal right breast. Craniocaudal image from a ductogram

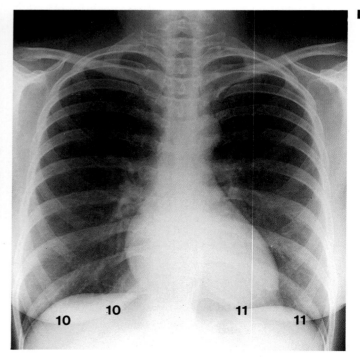

D Breasts of an adult female. Postero-anterior projection

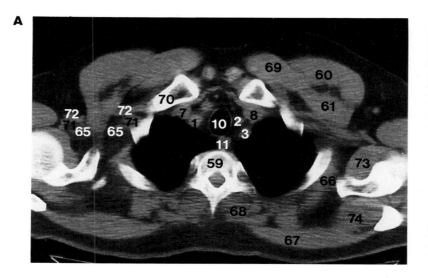

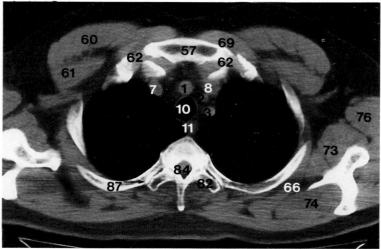

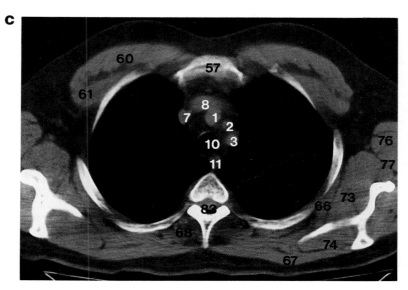

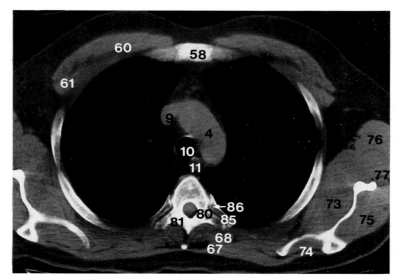

A–R Chest. Axial CT images **A–D** Mediastinal window settings

1	Brachiocephalic trunk	29	Right ⎫ inferior pulmonary vein	56	Internal thoracic artery and vein	85	Head ⎫ of rib
2	Left common carotid artery	30	Left ⎭	57	Manubrium ⎫ of sternum	86	Joint of head ⎭
3	Left subclavian artery	31	Right ⎫ coronary artery	58	Body ⎭	87	Costotransverse joint
4	Arch of aorta (aortic knuckle or knob)	32	Left ⎭	59	Body of vertebra	88	Plane of oblique fissure
5	Ascending ⎫ aorta	33	Anterior interventricular ⎫ branch of left coronary artery	60	Pectoralis major muscle	89	Middle lobe ⎫ segmental bronchus
6	Descending ⎭	34	Circumflex ⎭	61	Pectoralis minor muscle	90	Lingular ⎭
7	Right ⎫ brachiocephalic vein	35	Right ⎫ atrial appendage (auricle)	62	Sternoclavicular joint	91	Apical segment ⎫ inferior lobe
8	Left ⎭	36	Left ⎭	63	Axillary artery	92	Basal segment ⎭ bronchus
9	Superior vena cava	37	Right ⎫ atrium	64	Axillary vein	93	Anterior segment ⎫ superior
10	Trachea	38	Left ⎭	65	Brachial plexus	94	Posterior segment ⎭ lobe
11	Oesophagus	39	Interatrial septum	66	Serratus anterior muscle	95	Medial segment ⎫ middle lobe
12	Carina (bifurcation of trachea)	40	Cusp (leaflet) of tricuspid valve	67	Trapezius muscle	96	Lateral segment ⎭
13	Right ⎫ main bronchus	41	Cusp (leaflet) of mitral valve	68	Erector spinae muscle	97	Superior ⎫ lingular segment
14	Left ⎭	42	Chordae tendineae	69	Sternocleidomastoid muscle	98	Inferior ⎭
15	Right ⎫ superior lobe bronchus	43	Right ventricular wall	70	Clavicle	99	Apical segment ⎫ inferior lobe
16	Left ⎭	44	Right ventricular cavity	71	Right subclavian artery	100	Basal segment ⎭
17	Right ⎫ inferior lobe bronchus	45	Muscular ⎫ interventricular	72	Right subclavian vein	101	Right and left parietal pleura (anterior junctional line)
18	Left ⎭	46	Membranous ⎭ septum	73	Subscapularis muscle	102	Right common carotid artery
19	Right ⎫ superior intercostal vein	47	Fossa ovalis	74	Supraspinatus muscle	103	Vertebral artery
20	Left ⎭	48	Left ventricular wall	75	Infraspinatus muscle	104	Internal jugular vein
21	Azygos vein	49	Left ventricular cavity	76	Latissimus dorsi muscle	105	Thyroid lobe
22	Hemi-azygos vein	50	Papillary muscle	77	Teres major muscle		
23	Right ⎫ pulmonary artery	51	Coronary sinus	78	Teres minor muscle		
24	Left ⎭	52	Inferior vena cava	79	Rhomboid major muscle		
25	Superior lobe branch of right pulmonary artery	53	Posterior interventricular branch of right coronary artery	80	Pedicle		
26	Pulmonary trunk	54	Pericardium	81	Lamina		
27	Right ⎫ superior pulmonary vein	55	Pericardial recess	82	Transverse process		
28	Left ⎭			83	Vertebral foramen		
				84	Spinal cord		

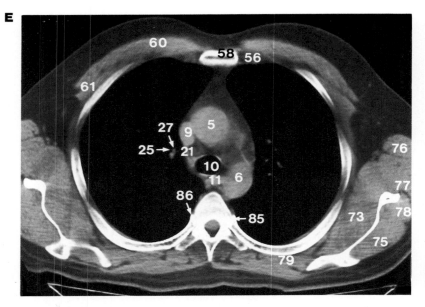

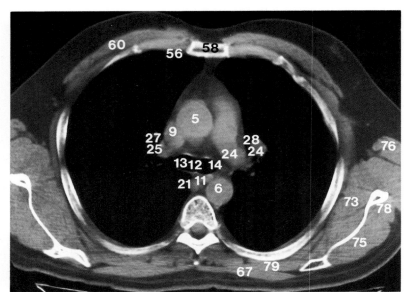

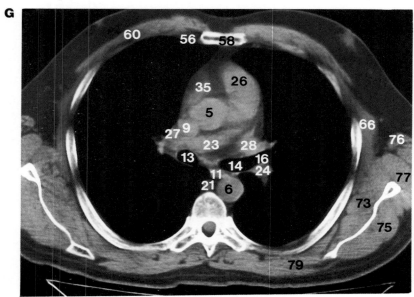

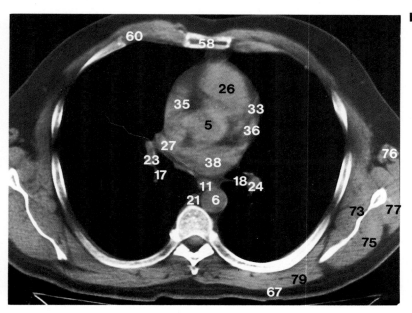

E–H Mediastinal window settings

1	Brachiocephalic trunk	19	Right ⎫ superior intercostal vein	37	Right ⎫ atrium	
2	Left common carotid artery	20	Left ⎭	38	Left ⎭	
3	Left subclavian artery	21	Azygos vein	39	Interatrial septum	
4	Arch of aorta (aortic knuckle or knob)	22	Hemi-azygos vein	40	Cusp (leaflet) of tricuspid valve	
5	Ascending ⎫ aorta	23	Right ⎫ pulmonary artery	41	Cusp (leaflet) of mitral valve	
6	Descending ⎭	24	Left ⎭	42	Chordae tendineae	
7	Right ⎫ brachiocephalic vein	25	Superior lobe branch of right pulmonary artery	43	Right ventricular wall	
8	Left ⎭	26	Pulmonary trunk	44	Right ventricular cavity	
9	Superior vena cava	27	Right ⎫ superior pulmonary vein	45	Muscular ⎫ interventricular	
10	Trachea	28	Left ⎭	46	Membranous ⎭ septum	
11	Oesophagus	29	Right ⎫ inferior pulmonary vein	47	Fossa ovalis	
12	Carina (bifurcation of trachea)	30	Left ⎭	48	Left ventricular wall	
13	Right ⎫ main bronchus	31	Right ⎫ coronary artery	49	Left ventricular cavity	
14	Left ⎭	32	Left ⎭	50	Papillary muscle	
15	Right ⎫ superior lobe bronchus	33	Anterior interventricular ⎫ branch of left	51	Coronary sinus	
16	Left ⎭	34	Circumflex ⎭ coronary artery	52	Inferior vena cava	
17	Right ⎫ inferior lobe bronchus	35	Right ⎫ atrial appendage (auricle)	53	Posterior interventricular branch of right coronary artery	
18	Left ⎭	36	Left ⎭			

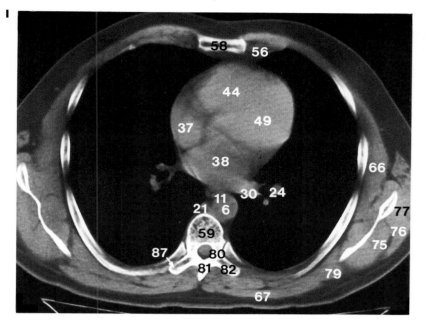
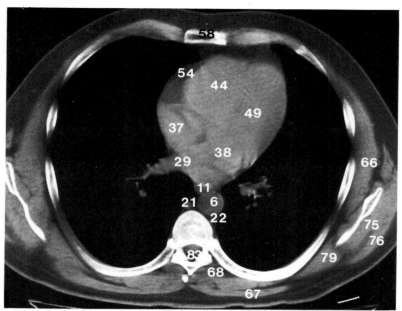
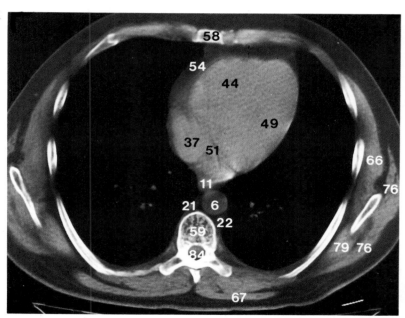
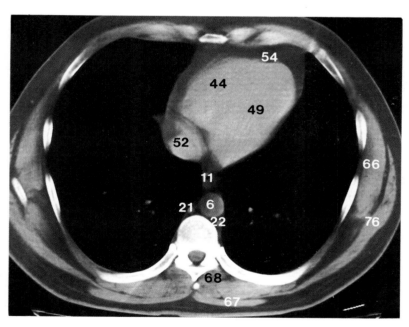

I–L Mediastinal window settings

54	Pericardium	71	Right subclavian artery	89	Middle lobe ⎫		
55	Pericardial recess	72	Right subclavian vein	90	Lingular ⎬ segmental bronchus		
56	Internal thoracic artery and vein	73	Subscapularis muscle	91	Apical segment ⎫		
		74	Supraspinatus muscle	92	Basal segment ⎬ inferior lobe bronchus		
57	Manubrium ⎫ of sternum	75	Infraspinatus muscle	93	Anterior segment ⎫		
58	Body ⎬	76	Latissimus dorsi muscle	94	Posterior segment ⎬ superior lobe		
59	Body of vertebra	77	Teres major muscle	95	Medial segment ⎫		
60	Pectoralis major muscle	78	Teres minor muscle	96	Lateral segment ⎬ middle lobe		
61	Pectoralis minor muscle	79	Rhomboid major muscle	97	Superior ⎫		
62	Sternoclavicular joint	80	Pedicle	98	Inferior ⎬ lingular segment		
63	Axillary artery	81	Lamina	99	Apical segment ⎫		
64	Axillary vein	82	Transverse process	100	Basal segment ⎬ inferior lobe		
65	Brachial plexus	83	Vertebral foramen	101	Right and left parietal pleura (anterior junctional line)		
66	Serratus anterior muscle	84	Spinal cord				
67	Trapezius muscle	85	Head ⎫ of rib	102	Right common carotid artery		
68	Erector spinae muscle	86	Joint of head ⎬	103	Vertebral artery		
69	Sternocleidomastoid muscle	87	Costotransverse joint	104	Internal jugular vein		
70	Clavicle	88	Plane of oblique fissure	105	Thyroid lobe		

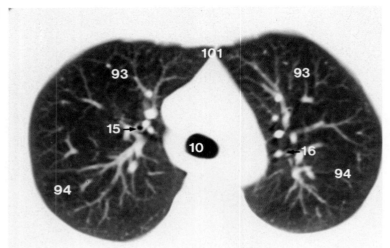

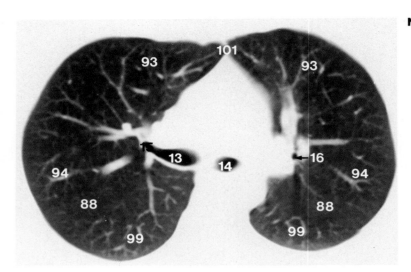

M—O Lung window settings

1	Brachiocephalic trunk
2	Left common carotid artery
3	Left subclavian artery
4	Arch of aorta (aortic knuckle or knob)
5	Ascending ⎫ aorta
6	Descending ⎭
7	Right ⎫ brachiocephalic vein
8	Left ⎭
9	Superior vena cava
10	Trachea
11	Oesophagus
12	Carina (bifurcation of trachea)
13	Right ⎫ main bronchus
14	Left ⎭
15	Right ⎫ superior lobe bronchus
16	Left ⎭
17	Right ⎫ inferior lobe bronchus
18	Left ⎭
19	Right ⎫ superior intercostal vein
20	Left ⎭
21	Azygos vein
22	Hemi-azygos vein
23	Right ⎫ pulmonary artery
24	Left ⎭
25	Superior lobe branch of right pulmonary artery
26	Pulmonary trunk
27	Right ⎫ superior pulmonary vein
28	Left ⎭
29	Right ⎫ inferior pulmonary vein
30	Left ⎭
31	Right ⎫ coronary artery
32	Left ⎭
33	Anterior interventricular ⎫ branch of left coronary
34	Circumflex ⎭ artery
35	Right ⎫ atrial appendage (auricle)
36	Left ⎭
37	Right ⎫ atrium
38	Left ⎭
39	Interatrial septum
40	Cusp (leaflet) of tricuspid valve
41	Cusp (leaflet) of mitral valve
42	Chordae tendineae
43	Right ventricular wall
44	Right ventricular cavity
45	Muscular ⎫ interventricular septum
46	Membranous ⎭
47	Fossa ovalis
48	Left ventricular wall
49	Left ventricular cavity
50	Papillary muscle
51	Coronary sinus

52	Inferior vena cava	79	Rhomboid major muscle
53	Posterior interventricular branch of right coronary artery	80	Pedicle
		81	Lamina
54	Pericardium	82	Transverse process
55	Pericardial recess	83	Vertebral foramen
56	Internal thoracic artery and vein	84	Spinal cord
57	Manubrium ⎫ of sternum	85	Head ⎫ of rib
58	Body ⎭	86	Joint of head ⎭
59	Body of vertebra	87	Costotransverse joint
60	Pectoralis major muscle	88	Plane of oblique fissure
61	Pectoralis minor muscle	89	Middle lobe ⎫ segmental
62	Sternoclavicular joint	90	Lingular ⎭ bronchus
63	Axillary artery	91	Apical segment ⎫ inferior lobe
64	Axillary vein	92	Basal segment ⎭ bronchus
65	Brachial plexus	93	Anterior segment ⎫ superior
66	Serratus anterior muscle	94	Posterior segment ⎭ lobe
67	Trapezius muscle	95	Medial segment ⎫ middle lobe
68	Erector spinae muscle	96	Lateral segment ⎭
69	Sternocleidomastoid muscle	97	Superior ⎫ lingular segment
70	Clavicle	98	Inferior ⎭
71	Right subclavian artery	99	Apical segment ⎫ inferior lobe
72	Right subclavian vein	100	Basal segment ⎭
73	Subscapularis muscle	101	Right and left parietal pleura (anterior junctional line)
74	Supraspinatus muscle		
75	Infraspinatus muscle	102	Right common carotid artery
76	Latissimus dorsi muscle	103	Vertebral artery
77	Teres major muscle	104	Internal jugular vein
78	Teres minor muscle	105	Thyroid lobe

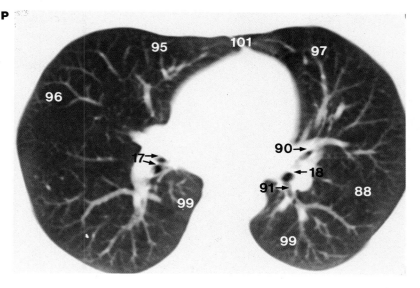

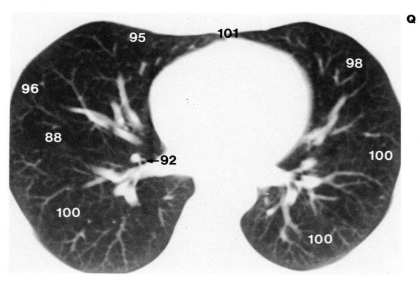

P–R Lung window settings

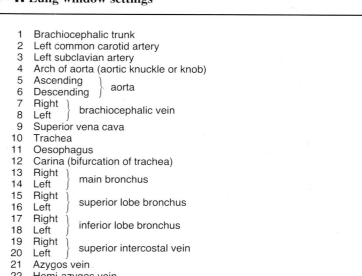

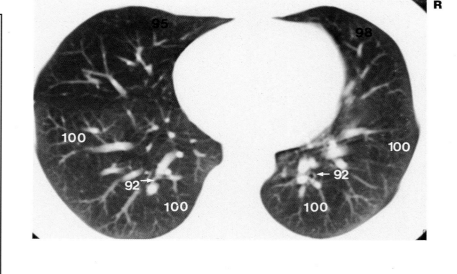

1 Brachiocephalic trunk
2 Left common carotid artery
3 Left subclavian artery
4 Arch of aorta (aortic knuckle or knob)
5 Ascending ⎫
6 Descending ⎬ aorta
7 Right ⎫
8 Left ⎬ brachiocephalic vein
9 Superior vena cava
10 Trachea
11 Oesophagus
12 Carina (bifurcation of trachea)
13 Right ⎫
14 Left ⎬ main bronchus
15 Right ⎫
16 Left ⎬ superior lobe bronchus
17 Right ⎫
18 Left ⎬ inferior lobe bronchus
19 Right ⎫
20 Left ⎬ superior intercostal vein
21 Azygos vein
22 Hemi-azygos vein
23 Right ⎫
24 Left ⎬ pulmonary artery
25 Superior lobe branch of right pulmonary artery
26 Pulmonary trunk
27 Right ⎫
28 Left ⎬ superior pulmonary vein
29 Right ⎫
30 Left ⎬ inferior pulmonary vein
31 Right ⎫
32 Left ⎬ coronary artery
33 Anterior interventricular ⎫ branch of left coronary
34 Circumflex ⎬ artery
35 Right ⎫
36 Left ⎬ atrial appendage (auricle)
37 Right ⎫
38 Left ⎬ atrium
39 Interatrial septum
40 Cusp (leaflet) of tricuspid valve
41 Cusp (leaflet) of mitral valve
42 Chordae tendineae
43 Right ventricular wall
44 Right ventricular cavity
45 Muscular ⎫
46 Membranous ⎬ interventricular septum
47 Fossa ovalis
48 Left ventricular wall
49 Left ventricular cavity
50 Papillary muscle
51 Coronary sinus

52 Inferior vena cava
53 Posterior interventricular branch of right coronary artery
54 Pericardium
55 Pericardial recess
56 Internal thoracic artery and vein
57 Manubrium ⎫
58 Body ⎬ of sternum
59 Body of vertebra
60 Pectoralis major muscle
61 Pectoralis minor muscle
62 Sternoclavicular joint
63 Axillary artery
64 Axillary vein
65 Brachial plexus
66 Serratus anterior muscle
67 Trapezius muscle
68 Erector spinae muscle
69 Sternocleidomastoid muscle
70 Clavicle
71 Right subclavian artery
72 Right subclavian vein
73 Subscapularis muscle
74 Supraspinatus muscle
75 Infraspinatus muscle
76 Latissimus dorsi muscle
77 Teres major muscle
78 Teres minor muscle

79 Rhomboid major muscle
80 Pedicle
81 Lamina
82 Transverse process
83 Vertebral foramen
84 Spinal cord
85 Head ⎫
86 Joint of head ⎬ of rib
87 Costotransverse joint
88 Plane of oblique fissure
89 Middle lobe ⎫ segmental
90 Lingular ⎬ bronchus
91 Apical segment ⎫ inferior lobe
92 Basal segment ⎬ bronchus
93 Anterior segment ⎫ superior
94 Posterior segment ⎬ lobe
95 Medial segment ⎫
96 Lateral segment ⎬ middle lobe
97 Superior ⎫
98 Inferior ⎬ lingular segment
99 Apical segment ⎫
100 Basal segment ⎬ inferior lobe
101 Right and left parietal pleura (anterior junctional line)
102 Right common carotid artery
103 Vertebral artery
104 Internal jugular vein
105 Thyroid lobe

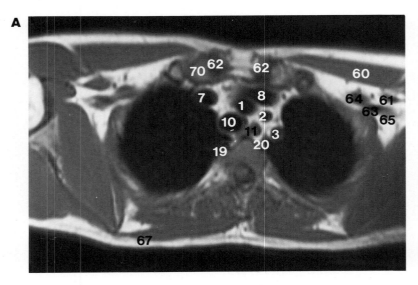

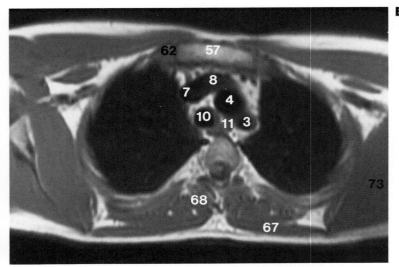

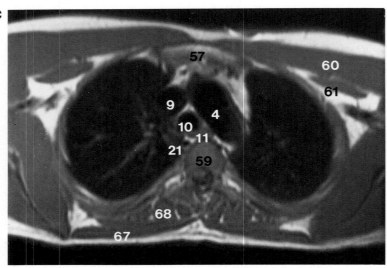

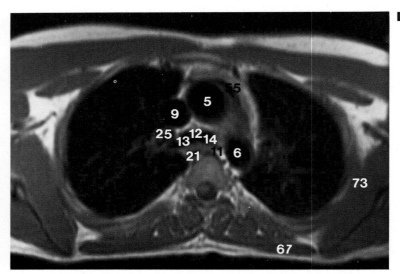

A—H Chest. Axial MR images (T$_1$-weighted)

1	Brachiocephalic trunk	19	Right	superior intercostal vein	37	Right atrium
2	Left common carotid artery	20	Left		38	Left
3	Left subclavian artery	21	Azygos vein		39	Interatrial septum
4	Arch of aorta (aortic knuckle or knob)	22	Hemi-azygos vein		40	Cusp (leaflet) of tricuspid valve
5	Ascending aorta	23	Right	pulmonary artery	41	Cusp (leaflet) of mitral valve
6	Descending aorta	24	Left		42	Chordae tendineae
7	Right brachiocephalic vein	25	Superior lobe branch of right pulmonary artery		43	Right ventricular wall
8	Left	26	Pulmonary trunk		44	Right ventricular cavity
9	Superior vena cava	27	Right	superior pulmonary vein	45	Muscular interventricular septum
10	Trachea	28	Left		46	Membranous
11	Oesophagus	29	Right	inferior pulmonary vein	47	Fossa ovalis
12	Carina (bifurcation of trachea)	30	Left		48	Left ventricular wall
13	Right main bronchus	31	Right	coronary artery	49	Left ventricular cavity
14	Left	32	Left		50	Papillary muscle
15	Right superior lobe bronchus	33	Anterior interventricular	branch of left coronary artery	51	Coronary sinus
16	Left	34	Circumflex		52	Inferior vena cava
17	Right inferior lobe bronchus	35	Right	atrial appendage (auricle)	53	Posterior interventricular branch of right coronary artery
18	Left	36	Left			

E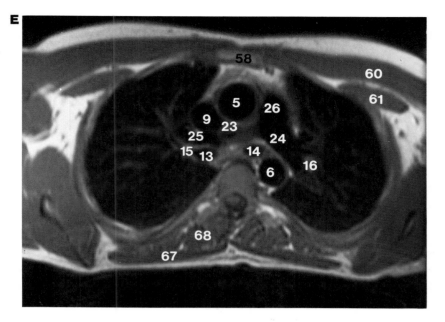

F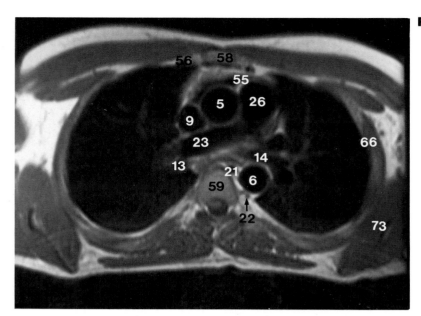

G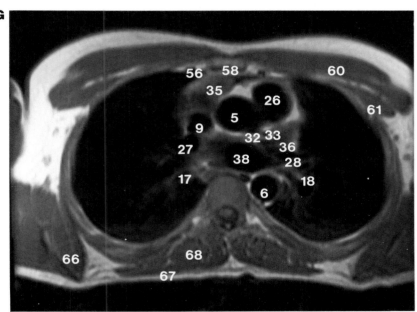

H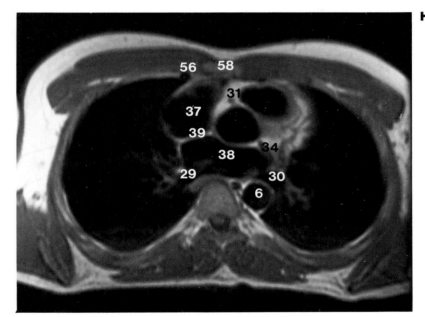

54	Pericardium	71	Right subclavian artery	89	Middle lobe } segmental bronchus
55	Pericardial recess	72	Right subclavian vein	90	Lingular
56	Internal thoracic artery and vein	73	Subscapularis muscle	91	Apical segment } inferior lobe bronchus
		74	Supraspinatus muscle	92	Basal segment
57	Manubrium } of sternum	75	Infraspinatus muscle	93	Anterior segment } superior lobe
58	Body	76	Latissimus dorsi muscle	94	Posterior segment
59	Body of vertebra	77	Teres major muscle	95	Medial segment } middle lobe
60	Pectoralis major muscle	78	Teres minor muscle	96	Lateral segment
61	Pectoralis minor muscle	79	Rhomboid major muscle	97	Superior } lingular segment
62	Sternoclavicular joint	80	Pedicle	98	Inferior
63	Axillary artery	81	Lamina	99	Apical segment } inferior lobe
64	Axillary vein	82	Transverse process	100	Basal segment
65	Brachial plexus	83	Vertebral foramen	101	Right and left parietal pleura (anterior junctional line)
66	Serratus anterior muscle	84	Spinal cord		
67	Trapezius muscle	85	Head } of rib	102	Right common carotid artery
68	Erector spinae muscle	86	Joint of head	103	Vertebral artery
69	Sternocleidomastoid muscle	87	Costotransverse joint	104	Internal jugular vein
70	Clavicle	88	Plane of oblique fissure	105	Thyroid lobe

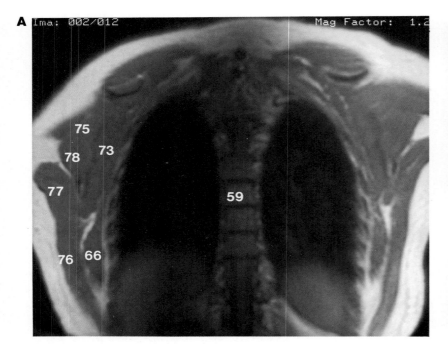

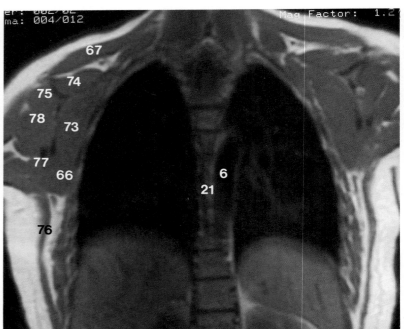

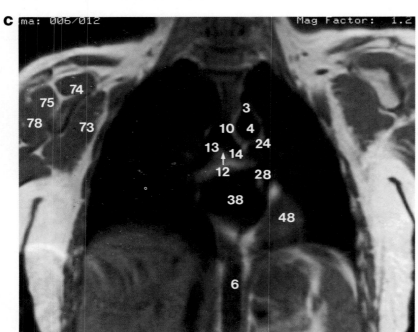

A–F Chest. Coronal MR images (T$_1$-weighted)

1	Brachiocephalic trunk	27	Right ⎫ superior pulmonary vein
2	Left common carotid artery	28	Left ⎭
3	Left subclavian artery	29	Right ⎫ inferior pulmonary vein
4	Arch of aorta (aortic knuckle or knob)	30	Left ⎭
5	Ascending ⎫ aorta	31	Right ⎫ coronary artery
6	Descending ⎭	32	Left ⎭
7	Right ⎫ brachiocephalic	33	Anterior interventricular ⎫ branch of left coronary artery
8	Left ⎭ vein	34	Circumflex ⎭
9	Superior vena cava	35	Right ⎫ atrial appendage
10	Trachea	36	Left ⎭ (auricle)
11	Oesophagus	37	Right ⎫ atrium
12	Carina (bifurcation of trachea)	38	Left ⎭
13	Right ⎫ main bronchus	39	Interatrial septum
14	Left ⎭	40	Cusp (leaflet) of tricuspid valve
15	Right ⎫ superior lobe	41	Cusp (leaflet) of mitral valve
16	Left ⎭ broncus	42	Chordae tendineae
17	Right ⎫ inferior lobe	43	Right ventricular wall
18	Left ⎭ bronchus	44	Right ventricular cavity
19	Right ⎫ superior intercostal	45	Muscular ⎫ interventricular
20	Left ⎭ vein	46	Membranous ⎭ septum
21	Azygos vein	47	Fossa ovalis
22	Hemi-azygos vein	48	Left ventricular wall
23	Right ⎫ pulmonary artery	49	Left ventricular cavity
24	Left ⎭	50	Papillary muscle
25	Superior lobe branch of right pulmonary artery	51	Coronary sinus
26	Pulmonary trunk	52	Inferior vena cava

D Ima: 007/012   Mag Factor: 1.2

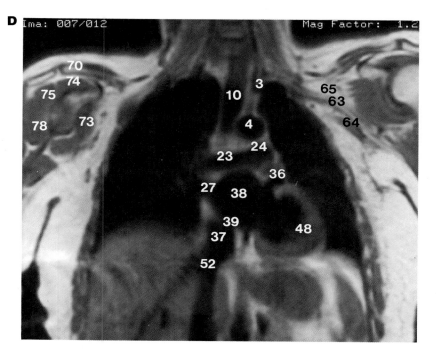

E Ima: 008/012   Mag Factor: 1.2

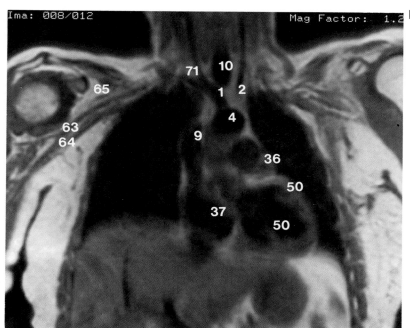

53	Posterior interventricular	79 Rhomboid major muscle

53 Posterior interventricular branch of right coronary artery
54 Pericardium
55 Pericardial recess
56 Internal thoracic artery and vein
57 Manubrium ⎱ of sternum
58 Body ⎰
59 Body of vertebra
60 Pectoralis major muscle
61 Pectoralis minor muscle
62 Sternoclavicular joint
63 Axillary artery
64 Axillary vein
65 Brachial plexus
66 Serratus anterior muscle
67 Trapezius muscle
68 Erector spinae muscle
69 Sternocleidomastoid muscle
70 Clavicle
71 Right subclavian artery
72 Right subclavian vein
73 Subscapularis muscle
74 Supraspinatus muscle
75 Infraspinatus muscle
76 Latissimus dorsi muscle
77 Teres major muscle
78 Teres minor muscle

79 Rhomboid major muscle
80 Pedicle
81 Lamina
82 Transverse process
83 Vertebral foramen
84 Spinal cord
85 Head ⎱ of rib
86 Joint of head ⎰
87 Costotransverse joint
88 Plane of oblique fissure
89 Middle lobe ⎱ segmental
90 Lingular ⎰ bronchus
91 Apical segment ⎱ inferior lobe
92 Basal segment ⎰ bronchus
93 Anterior segment ⎱ superior
94 Posterior segment ⎰ lobe
95 Medial segment ⎱ middle lobe
96 Lateral segment ⎰
97 Superior ⎱ lingular segment
98 Inferior ⎰
99 Apical segment ⎱ inferior lobe
100 Basal segment ⎰
101 Right and left parietal pleura (anterior junctional line)
102 Right common carotid artery
103 Vertebral artery
104 Internal jugular vein
105 Thyroid lobe

F Std: 00423
Ser: 002/02
Ima: 009/012
Signa 1.3
A 26.3 m
Mag Factor: 1.2

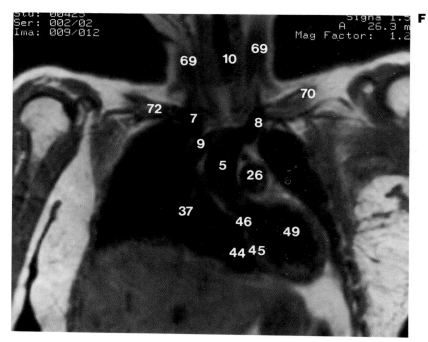

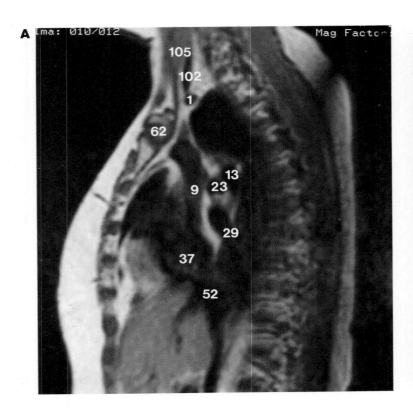

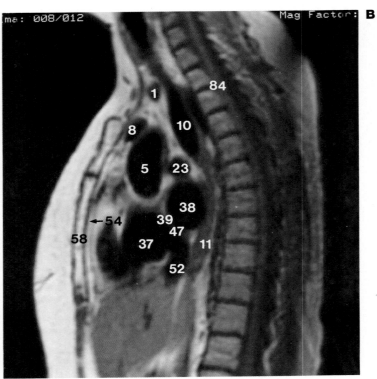

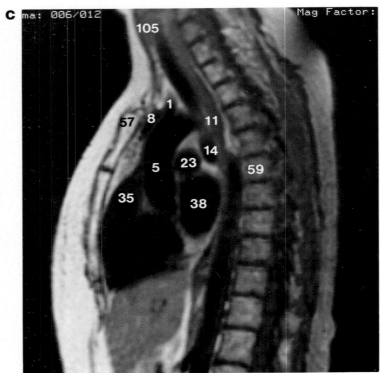

A—F Chest. Sagittal MR images (T$_1$-weighted)

1	Brachiocephalic trunk	27	Right ⎱ superior pulmonary vein
2	Left common carotid artery	28	Left ⎰
3	Left subclavian artery	29	Right ⎱ inferior pulmonary vein
4	Arch of aorta (aortic knuckle or knob)	30	Left ⎰
		31	Right ⎱ coronary artery
5	Ascending ⎱ aorta	32	Left ⎰
6	Descending ⎰	33	Anterior interventricular ⎱ branch of left
7	Right ⎱ brachiocephalic vein		Circumflex ⎰ coronary artery
8	Left ⎰	34	Circumflex
9	Superior vena cava	35	Right ⎱ atrial appendage
10	Trachea	36	Left ⎰ (auricle)
11	Oesophagus	37	Right ⎱ atrium
12	Carina (bifurcation of trachea)	38	Left ⎰
13	Right ⎱ main bronchus	39	Interatrial septum
14	Left ⎰	40	Cusp (leaflet) of tricuspid valve
15	Right ⎱ superior lobe		
16	Left ⎰ bronchus	41	Cusp (leaflet) of mitral valve
17	Right ⎱ inferior lobe	42	Chordae tendineae
18	Left ⎰ bronchus	43	Right ventricular wall
19	Right ⎱ superior intercostal	44	Right ventricular cavity
20	Left ⎰ vein	45	Muscular ⎱ interventricular
21	Azygos vein	46	Membranous ⎰ septum
22	Hemi-azygos vein	47	Fossa ovalis
23	Right ⎱ pulmonary artery	48	Left ventricular wall
24	Left ⎰	49	Left ventricular cavity
25	Superior lobe branch of right pulmonary artery	50	Papillary muscle
		51	Coronary sinus
26	Pulmonary trunk	52	Inferior vena cava

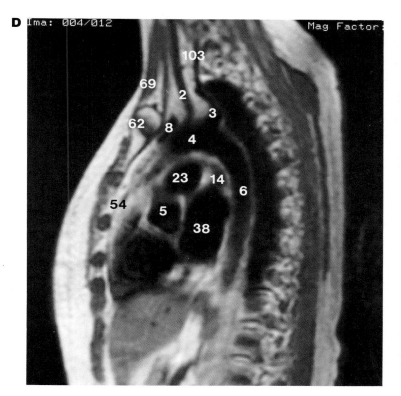

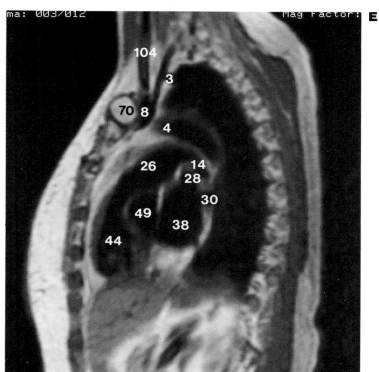

53	Posterior interventricular branch of right coronary artery	79	Rhomboid major muscle
		80	Pedicle
54	Pericardium	81	Lamina
55	Pericardial recess	82	Transverse process
56	Internal thoracic artery and vein	83	Vertebral foramen
		84	Spinal cord
57	Manubrium } of sternum	85	Head } of rib
58	Body	86	Joint of head
59	Body of vertebra	87	Costotransverse joint
60	Pectoralis major muscle	88	Plane of oblique fissure
61	Pectoralis minor muscle	89	Middle lobe } segmental
62	Sternoclavicular joint	90	Lingular } bronchus
63	Axillary artery	91	Apical segment } inferior lobe
64	Axillary vein	92	Basal segment } bronchus
65	Brachial plexus	93	Anterior segment } superior
66	Serratus anterior muscle	94	Posterior segment } lobe
67	Trapezius muscle	95	Medial segment } middle lobe
68	Erector spinae muscle	96	Lateral segment
69	Sternocleidomastoid muscle	97	Superior } lingular segment
70	Clavicle	98	Inferior
71	Right subclavian artery	99	Apical segment } inferior lobe
72	Right subclavian vein	100	Basal segment
73	Subscapularis muscle	101	Right and left parietal pleura (anterior junctional line)
74	Supraspinatus muscle	102	Right common carotid artery
75	Infraspinatus muscle	103	Vertebral artery
76	Latissimus dorsi muscle	104	Internal jugular vein
77	Teres major muscle	105	Thyroid lobe
78	Teres minor muscle		

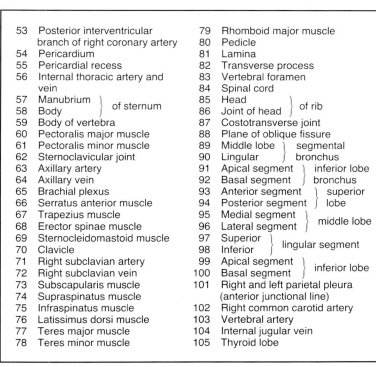

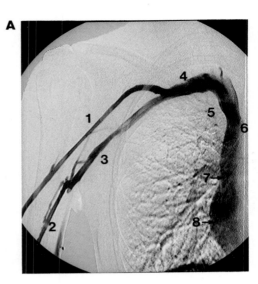

A Subtracted superior vena cavogram

1 Cephalic vein
2 Basilic vein
3 Axillary vein
4 Subclavian vein
5 Brachiocephalic vein
6 Site of entry of left brachiocephalic vein
7 Superior vena cava
8 Right atrium

B Pulmonary arteriogram

1 Catheter introduced via right brachial vein
2 Tip of catheter in main pulmonary artery
3 Right ⎫
4 Left ⎬ pulmonary artery
5 Superior lobe ⎫
6 Inferior lobe ⎬ pulmonary artery
7 Middle lobe ⎭
8 Lateral ⎫
9 Posterior ⎬ basal artery
10 Medial ⎭
11 Medial artery (middle lobe)
12 Lateral artery (middle lobe)
13 Apical artery (superior lobe)
14 Posterior artery (superior lobe)
15 Anterior artery (superior lobe)
16 Superior ⎫
17 Inferior ⎬ lingular artery

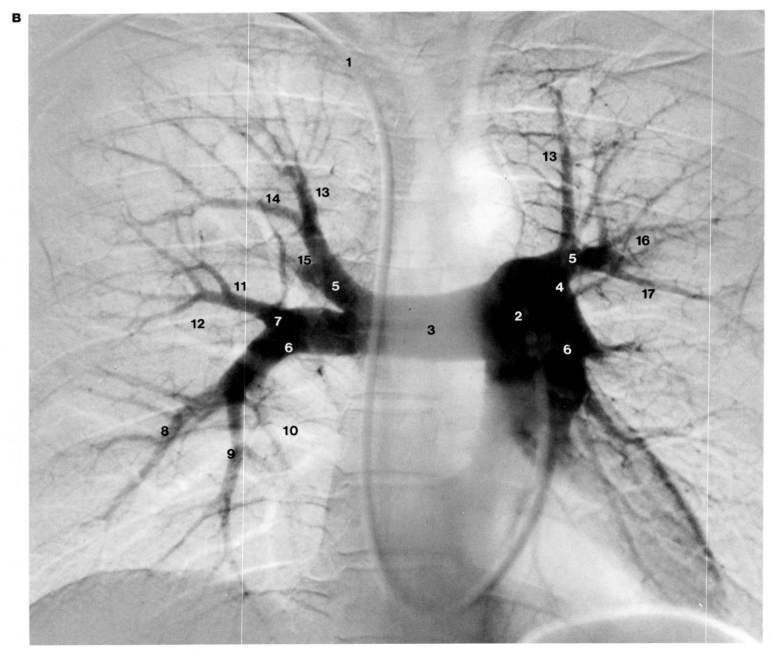

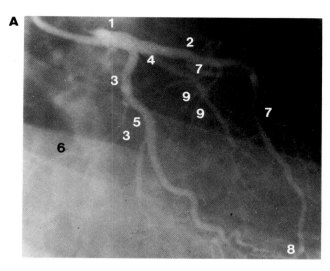

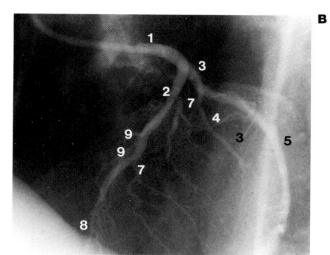

Left coronary arteriograms, A right anterior oblique image, **B** and **C** left anterior oblique images, **D** lateral image

1 Left main stem coronary artery
2 Left anterior interventricular branch (left anterior descending)
3 Circumflex artery
4 First ⎫ obtuse marginal
5 Second ⎭ branch of circumflex artery
6 Branch to left atrium
7 Diagonal arteries
8 Left anterior interventricular artery curving round apex of heart
9 Septal arteries

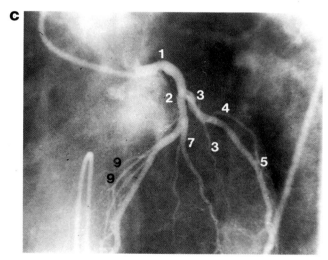

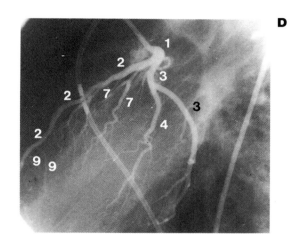

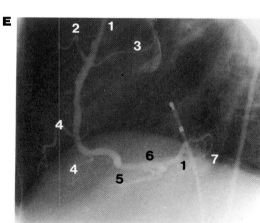

E and **F Right coronary arteriograms. Lateral images**

1 Right coronary artery
2 Conus artery
3 Sinuatrial nodal artery
4 Right marginal arteries
5 Posterior interventricular septal artery (posterior descending artery)
6 Atrioventricular nodal artery
7 Lateral ventricular branch to left ventricle
8 Branch to left atrium
9 Septal arteries

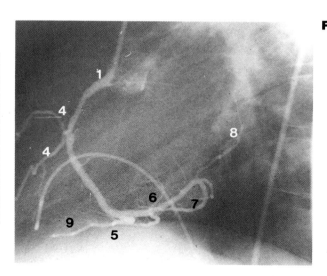

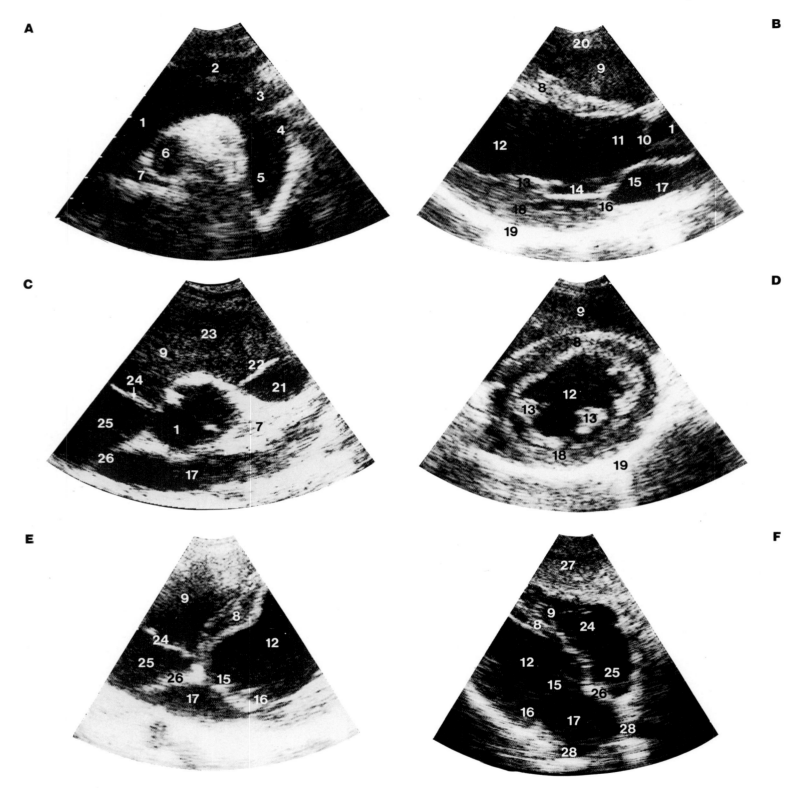

Heart, **A** suprasternal arch of aorta, **B** left parasternal long axis of left ventricle, **C** left parasternal short axis at aortic valve, **D** left parasternal short axis at papillary muscles, **E** apical four chamber, **F** subcostal four chamber. Ultrasound images

1	Ascending aorta	8	Interventricular septum	15	Anterior ⎫ cusp of mitral valve	22	Pulmonary valve
2	Brachiocephalic trunk	9	Right ventricle	16	Posterior ⎭	23	Right ventricular outflow tract
3	Left common carotid artery	10	Aortic valve	17	Left atrium	24	Tricuspid valve
4	Left subclavian artery	11	Left ventricular outflow tract	18	Myocardium	25	Right atrium
5	Descending thoracic aorta	12	Left ventricle	19	Pericardium	26	Interatrial septum
6	Left pulmonary artery	13	Papillary muscles	20	Anterior wall of right ventricle	27	Left lobe of liver
7	Left coronary artery	14	Chordae tendineae	21	Pulmonary artery	28	Pulmonary vein

A Subtracted arch aortogram.
Anteroposterior image

1	Ascending aorta
2	Brachiocephalic trunk
3	Left common carotid artery
4	Left subclavian artery
5	Right subclavian artery
6	Right common carotid artery
7	Vertebral artery
8	Internal thoracic artery
9	Inferior thyroid artery
10	Ascending cervical artery
11	Thyrocervical trunk
12	Suprascapular artery
13	Costocervical trunk
14	Superior thoracic artery
15	Lateral thoracic artery
16	Deltoid branch of thoraco-acromial artery

● The vertebral artery (7) has a separate origin off the arch, projected over the left common carotid artery in this view. This is a normal variant.

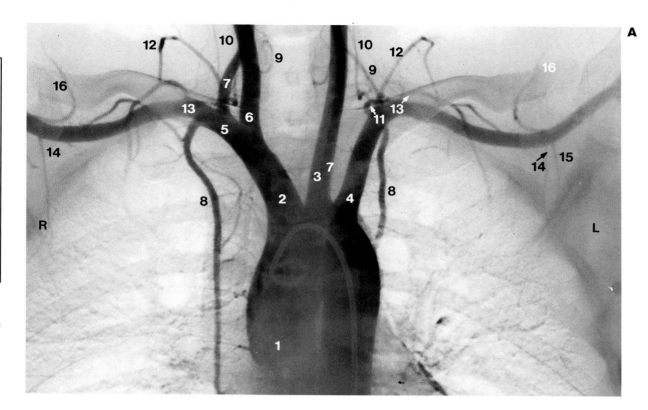

B Subtracted arch aortogram.
Left anterior oblique image

The origins of the supra-aortic branches are best shown by left anterior oblique projection, so that the origins of the vessels are not superimposed. There are many congenital variations in the way in which the major vessels arise from the aortic arch, but the most common is shown in **B**.

1	Ascending aorta
2	Brachiocephalic trunk
3	Left common carotid artery
4	Left subclavian artery
5	Right subclavian artery
6	Right common carotid artery
7	Vertebral artery
8	Internal thoracic artery
9	Inferior thyroid artery
10	Ascending cervical artery
11	Thyrocervical trunk
12	Costocervical trunk
13	Intercostal artery

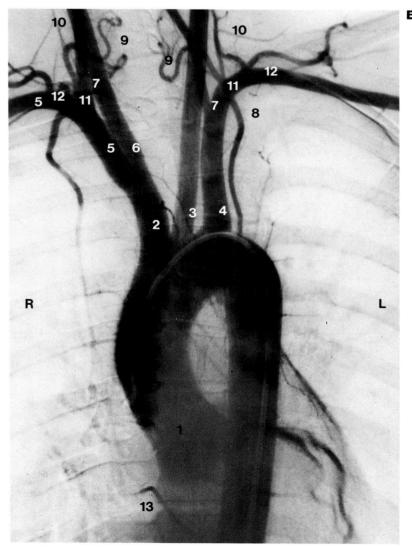

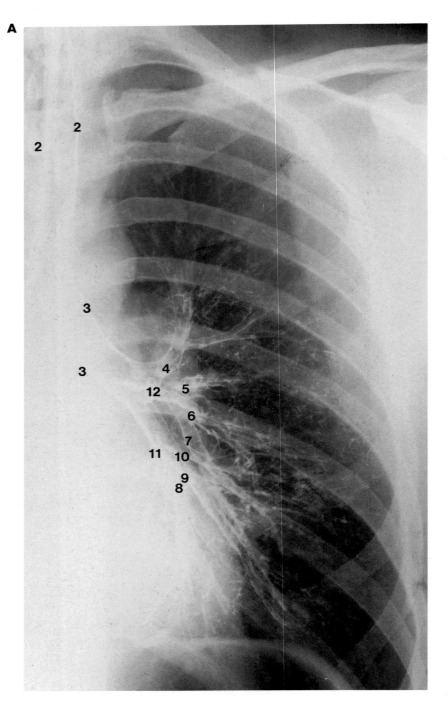

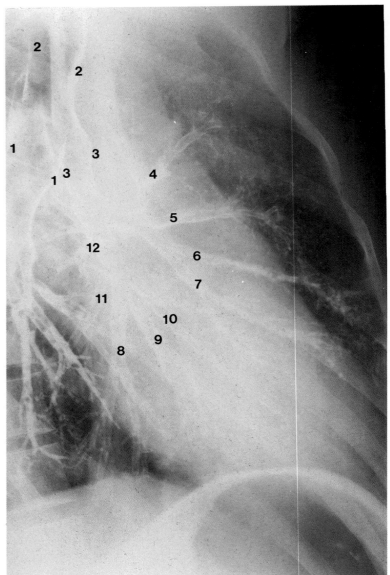

Left lung bronchogram, A postero-anterior image, B oblique image

1	Right main bronchus	8	Posterior
2	Trachea	9	Lateral — basal segmental
3	Left main bronchus	10	Anterior — bronchus
4	Apicoposterior segmental bronchus	11	Medial
5	Anterior segmental bronchus	12	Apical (superior) segmental
6	Superior — lingular segmental		bronchus
7	Inferior — bronchus		

A

B

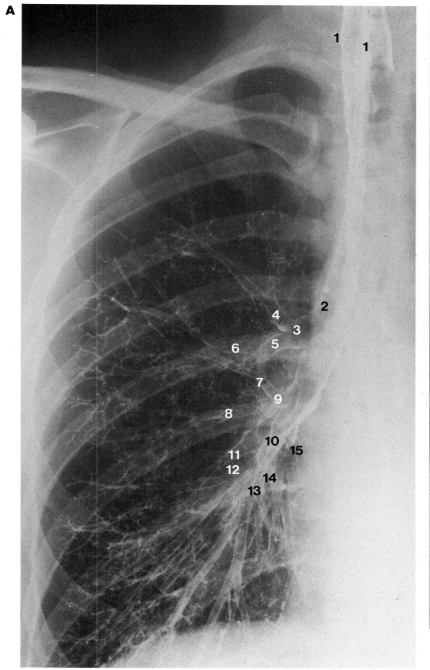
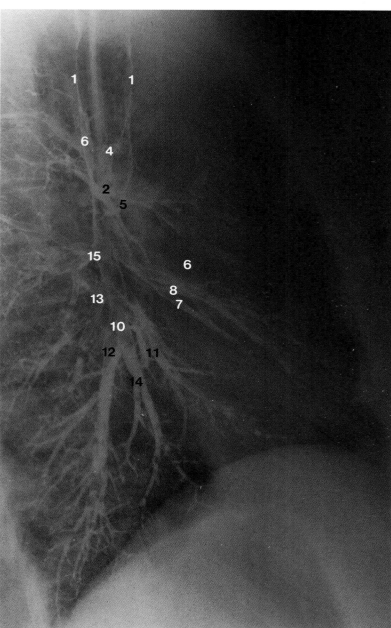

Right lung bronchogram, A postero-anterior image, B lateral image

1	Trachea	7	Medial segmental bronchus } of middle lobe	11	Anterior }
2	Right main bronchus	8	Lateral segmental bronchus }	12	Lateral } basal segmental bronchus
3	Right superior lobe bronchus	9	Middle } lobe bronchus	13	Posterior }
4	Apical }	10	Inferior }	14	Medial }
5	Anterior } segmental bronchus			15	Apical (superior) segmental bronchus
6	Posterior }				

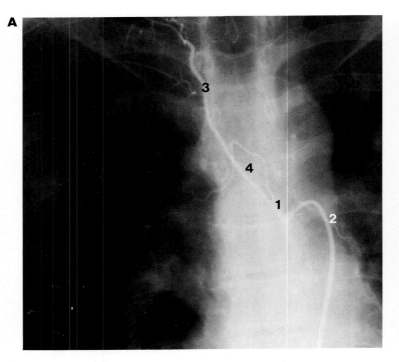

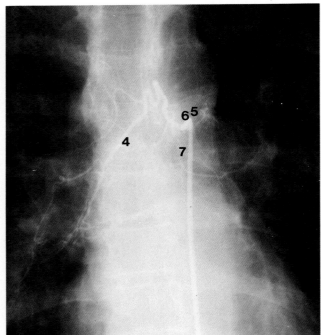

A and B Right bronchial arteriograms

There is great variability in the anatomy of the bronchial arteries, but the majority originate from the descending thoracic aorta, above the level of the left main stem bronchus between the upper border of the fifth thoracic vertebra and the lower border of the sixth thoracic vertebra. The number of bronchial arteries on each side may vary between one and four. Usually, there is one vessel to the right lung and two to the left. Accessory bronchial arteries may arise from the brachiocephalic artery and subclavian arteries, or from other branches such as the internal thoracic, pericardiophrenic and oesophageal arteries. In many cases the right bronchial artery arises from an intercostobronchial trunk, but in this example the trunk is very short and divides almost immediately into a right bronchial artery, which is directed towards the hilum, and the first right aortic intercostal artery. Reflux filling of the left bronchial artery is seen.

A second larger bronchial artery has been catheterised (**B**) which has a common trunk arising from the front of the aorta, giving rise to a right and left bronchial artery.

1	Tip of catheter in intercostobronchial trunk
2	Reflux filling of left bronchial artery
3	Intercostal artery
4	Right bronchial artery
5	Tip of catheter in common bronchial arterial trunk
6	Common bronchial trunk
7	Left bronchial branches

C Azygos venogram

In the thorax the vertebral veins drain into intercostal veins, while in the lumbar region the lumbar veins drain into the ascending lumbar veins. The right ascending lumbar vein becomes the azygos vein on entering the thorax, and the left ascending lumbar vein becomes the hemi-azygos vein. At the level of the fourth thoracic vertebra, the azygos vein turns anteriorly (the arch of the azygos) to enter the superior vena cava. The hemiazygos vein crosses to join the azygos vein at the level of the eighth or ninth thoracic vertebral body. The accessory hemi-azygos vein is continuous with the hemi-azygos vein inferiorly and the left superior intercostal vein superiorly.

1	Tip of catheter introduced via femoral vein into superior vena cava and azygos vein
2	Subtraction artefact caused by cardiac and catheter movement
3	Azygos arch
4	Azygos vein
5	Intercostal veins
6	Accessory hemi-azygos vein
7	Hemi-azygos vein

Abdomen

Abdomen. Supine projection

1 Right kidney
2 Gas in stomach
3 Left kidney
4 Gas in descending colon
5 Left ⎫
6 Right ⎬ psoas muscle
7 Gas in caecum and
   ascending colon

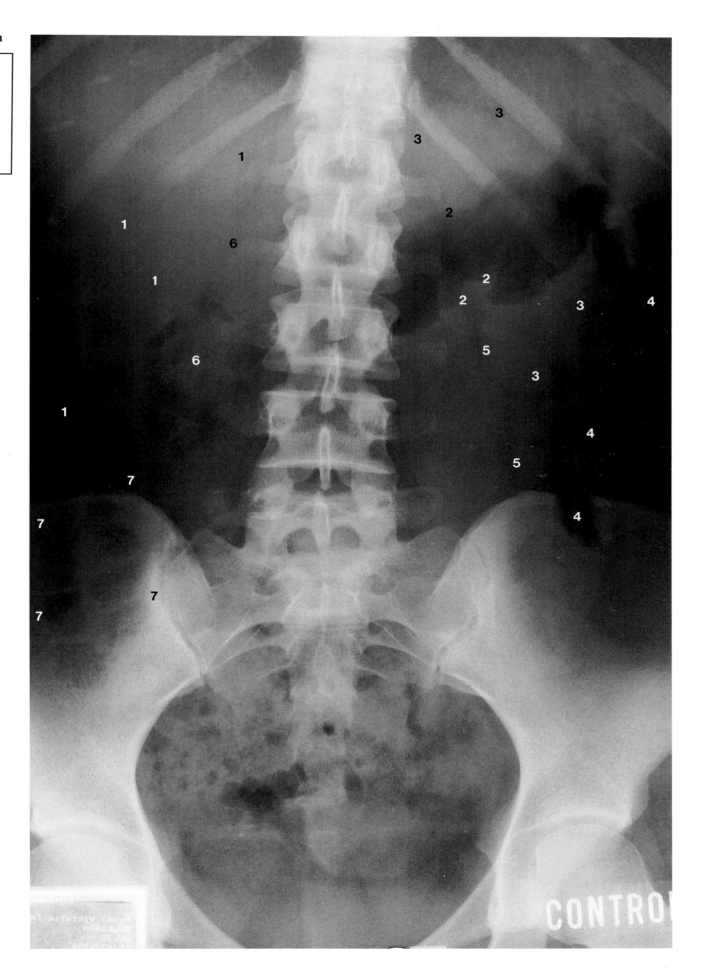

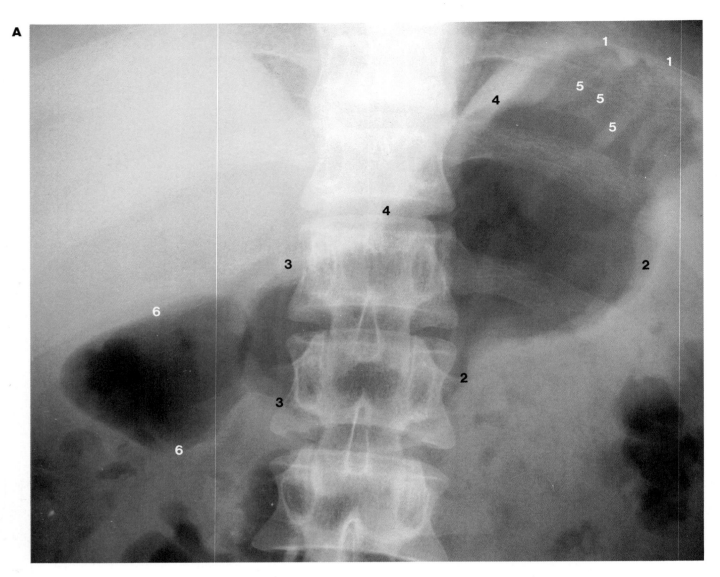

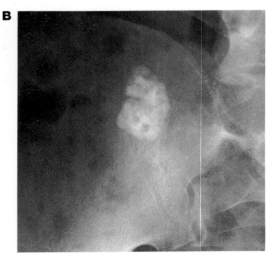

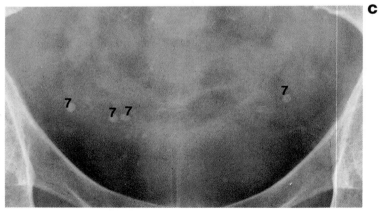

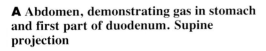

A Abdomen, demonstrating gas in stomach and first part of duodenum. Supine projection

Abdomen, **B** demonstrating a calcified lymph node, **C** demonstrating calcified pelvic veins (phleboliths). Supine projections

1 Fundus
2 Greater curvature ⎫
3 Antrum   ⎬ of stomach
4 Lesser curvature ⎭
5 Rugae
6 Superior (first) part of duodenum (duodenal cap)
7 Phlebolith

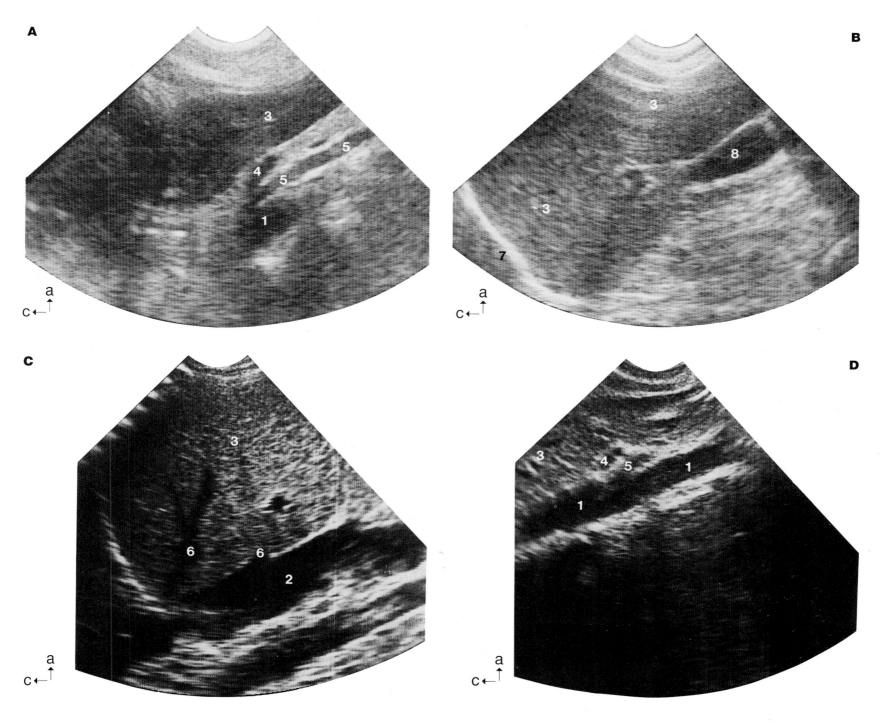

A–D Upper abdomen. Parasagittal ultrasound images (a = anterior, c = cranial)

1	Abdominal aorta
2	Inferior vena cava
3	Liver
4	Coeliac trunk
5	Superior mesenteric artery
6	Hepatic veins
7	Right hemidiaphragm
8	Gall bladder

111

A

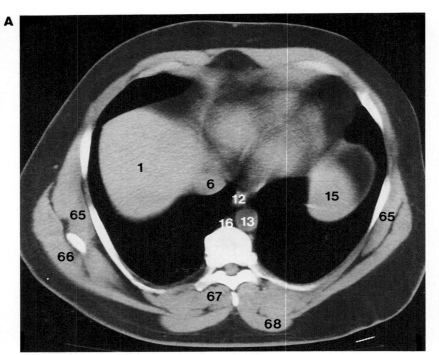

B

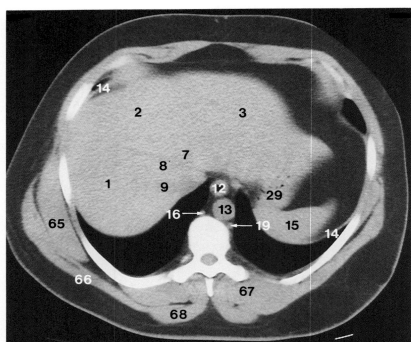

C

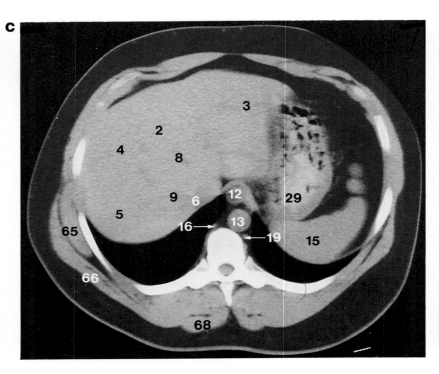

D

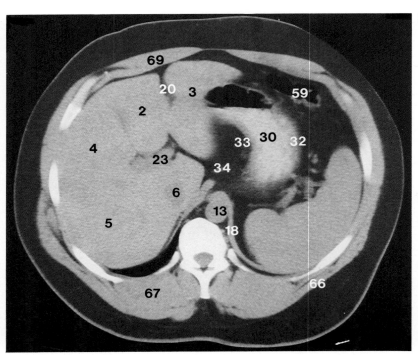

A—K Abdomen. Axial CT images

1	Right lobe	13	Aorta	25 Common bile duct	37 Splenic artery
2	Medial segment of left lobe	14	Diaphragm	26 Gall bladder	38 Splenic vein
3	Lateral segment of left lobe	15	Spleen	27 Caudate lobe of liver	39 Superior mesenteric artery
4	Anterior segment of right lobe	16	Azygos vein	28 Gastro-oesophageal junction	40 Superior mesenteric vein
5	Posterior segment of right lobe	17	Right } crus of diaphragm	29 Fundus	41 Tail
6	Inferior vena cava	18	Left	30 Body } of stomach	42 Body } of pancreas
7	Left	19	Hemi-azygos vein	31 Pyloric part	43 Neck
8	Middle } hepatic vein	20	Fissure for ligamentum venosum	32 Greater curvature	44 Head
9	Right	21	Porta hepatis	33 Lesser curvature	45 Uncinate process of head
10	Right } ventricle	22	Coeliac trunk	34 Left gastric artery	46 Superior (first) } part of duodenum
11	Left	23	Portal vein	35 Right } suprarenal gland	47 Descending (second)
12	Oesophagus	24	Hepatic artery	36 Left	48 Horizontal (third)

Legend column groupings:
- 1–5: of liver
- 17, 18: crus of diaphragm
- 29–33: of stomach
- 35, 36: suprarenal gland
- 41–45: of pancreas
- 46–48: part of duodenum

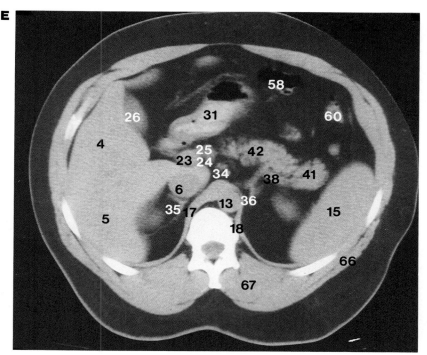

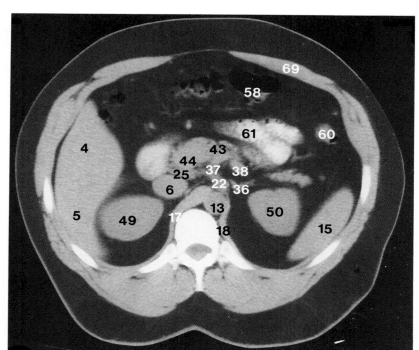

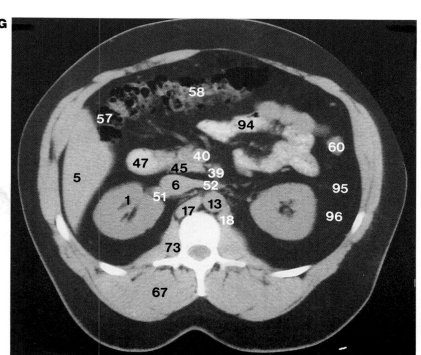

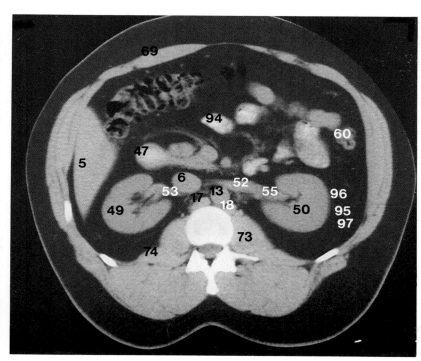

49	Right	} kidney	62	Falciform ligament	75	Inferior mesenteric vein	88	Ureter
50	Left		63	Body	} of sternum	76	Inferior mesenteric artery	89	Gluteus maximus muscle
51	Right	} renal vein	64	Xiphoid process		77	Right	} atrium	90	Iliotibial tract
52	Left		65	Serratus anterior muscle	78	Left	91	Internal iliac artery
53	Right	} renal artery	66	Latissimus dorsi muscle	79	Common iliac artery	92	Superior gluteal artery
54	Left		67	Erector spinae muscle	80	Common iliac vein	93	Gonadal artery and vein
55	Renal pelvis		68	Trapezius muscle	81	Body of vertebra	94	Ileum
56	Ascending colon		69	Rectus abdominis muscle	82	Intervertebral disc	95	Renal fascia
57	Right colic (hepatic) flexure		70	External oblique muscle	83	Thecal sac	96	Perirenal	} fat
58	Transverse colon		71	Internal oblique muscle	84	Ilium	97	Pararenal	
59	Left colic (splenic) flexure		72	Transversus abdominis muscle	85	Lateral part (ala) of sacrum		
60	Descending colon		73	Psoas major muscle	86	Sacro-iliac joint		
61	Jejunum		74	Quadratus lumborum muscle	87	Gluteus medius muscle		

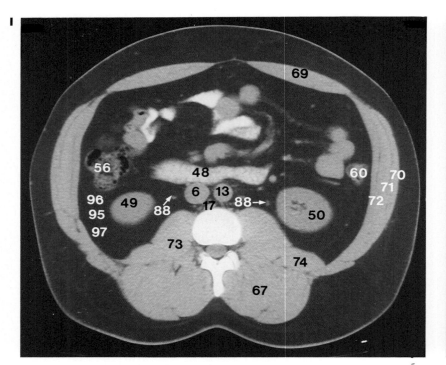

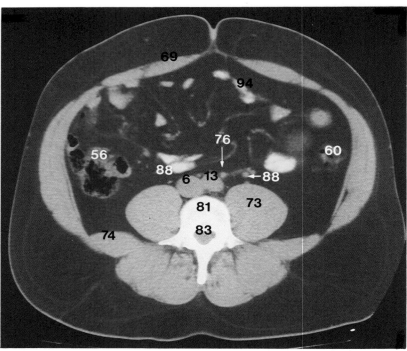

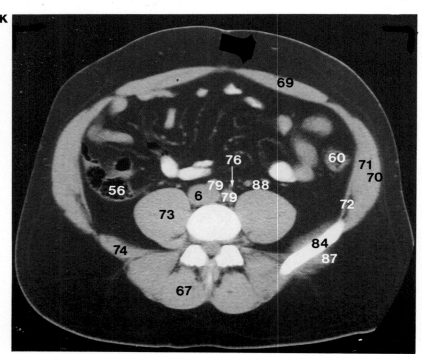

I–K Abdomen. Axial CT images

1	Right lobe		23	Portal vein	
2	Medial segment of left lobe		24	Hepatic artery	
3	Lateral segment of left lobe	of liver	25	Common bile duct	
4	Anterior segment of right lobe		26	Gall bladder	
5	Posterior segment of right lobe		27	Caudate lobe of liver	
			28	Gastro-oesophageal junction	
6	Inferior vena cava		29	Fundus	
7	Left		30	Body	of stomach
8	Middle	hepatic vein	31	Pyloric part	
9	Right		32	Greater curvature	
10	Right	ventricle	33	Lesser curvature	
11	Left		34	Left gastric artery	
12	Oesophagus		35	Right	suprarenal gland
13	Aorta		36	Left	
14	Diaphragm		37	Splenic artery	
15	Spleen		38	Splenic vein	
16	Azygos vein		39	Superior mesenteric artery	
17	Right	crus of diaphragm	40	Superior mesenteric vein	
18	Left		41	Tail	
19	Hemi-azygos vein		42	Body	of pancreas
20	Fissure for ligamentum venosum		43	Neck	
			44	Head	
21	Porta hepatis		45	Uncinate process of head	
22	Coeliac trunk		46	Superior (first)	part of duodenum
			47	Descending (second)	
			48	Horizontal (third)	

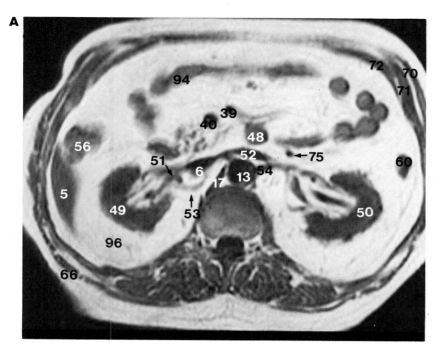

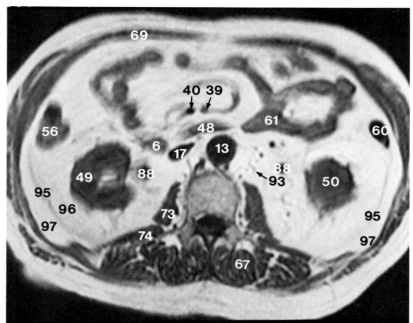

A—F Abdomen. Axial MR images (T₁-weighted)

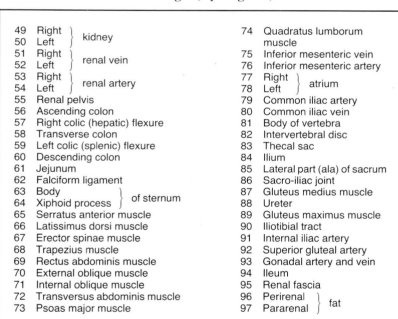

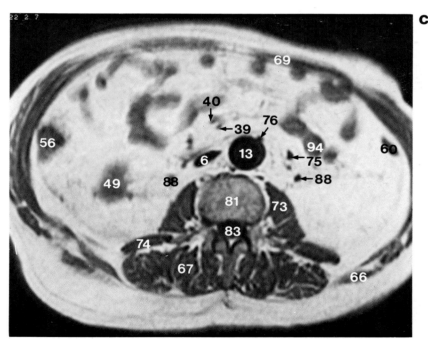

49	Right ⎫		74	Quadratus lumborum
50	Left ⎭ kidney			muscle
51	Right ⎫		75	Inferior mesenteric vein
52	Left ⎭ renal vein		76	Inferior mesenteric artery
53	Right ⎫		77	Right ⎫ atrium
54	Left ⎭ renal artery		78	Left ⎭
55	Renal pelvis		79	Common iliac artery
56	Ascending colon		80	Common iliac vein
57	Right colic (hepatic) flexure		81	Body of vertebra
58	Transverse colon		82	Intervertebral disc
59	Left colic (splenic) flexure		83	Thecal sac
60	Descending colon		84	Ilium
61	Jejunum		85	Lateral part (ala) of sacrum
62	Falciform ligament		86	Sacro-iliac joint
63	Body ⎫ of sternum		87	Gluteus medius muscle
64	Xiphoid process ⎭		88	Ureter
65	Serratus anterior muscle		89	Gluteus maximus muscle
66	Latissimus dorsi muscle		90	Iliotibial tract
67	Erector spinae muscle		91	Internal iliac artery
68	Trapezius muscle		92	Superior gluteal artery
69	Rectus abdominis muscle		93	Gonadal artery and vein
70	External oblique muscle		94	Ileum
71	Internal oblique muscle		95	Renal fascia
72	Transversus abdominis muscle		96	Perirenal ⎫ fat
73	Psoas major muscle		97	Pararenal ⎭

115

D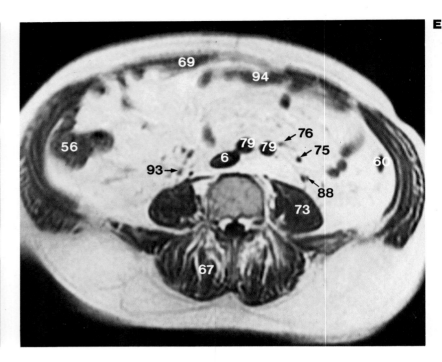

E

F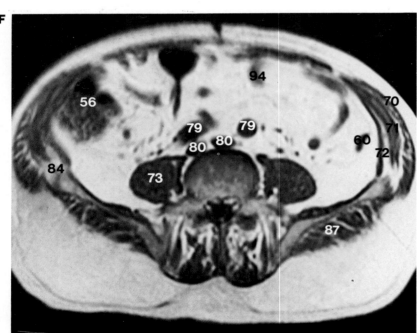

D–F Abdomen. Axial MR images (T$_1$-weighted)

1	Right lobe	21	Porta hepatis
2	Medial segment of left lobe	22	Coeliac trunk
3	Lateral segment of left lobe	23	Portal vein
		24	Hepatic artery
4	Anterior segment of right lobe	of liver	25	Common bile duct
		26	Gall bladder
5	Posterior segment of right lobe		27	Caudate lobe of liver
		28	Gastro-oesophageal junction
6	Inferior vena cava	29	Fundus
		30	Body
7	Left	hepatic vein	31	Pyloric part	of stomach
8	Middle		32	Greater curvature
9	Right		33	Lesser curvature
10	Right	ventricle	34	Left gastric artery
11	Left		35	Right	suprarenal gland
12	Oesophagus	36	Left
13	Aorta	37	Splenic artery
14	Diaphragm	38	Splenic vein
15	Spleen	39	Superior mesenteric artery
16	Azygos vein	40	Superior mesenteric vein
17	Right	crus of diaphragm	41	Tail
18	Left		42	Body
19	Hemi-azygos vein	43	Neck	of pancreas
20	Fissure for ligamentum venosum	44	Head
		45	Uncinate process of head

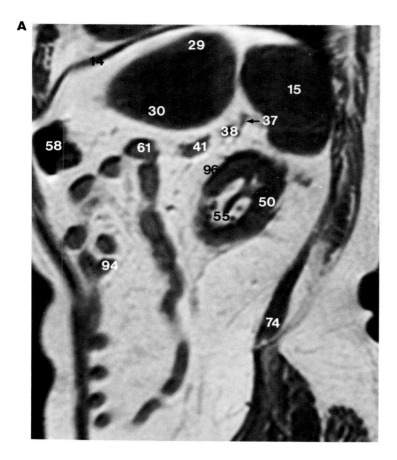

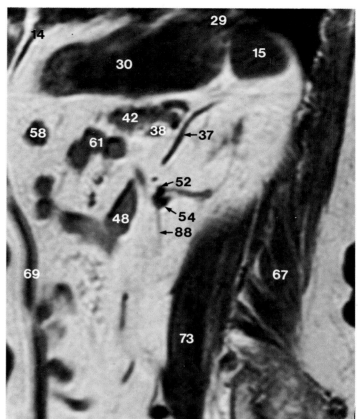

A—F Abdomen. Sagittal MR images (T$_1$-weighted)

46	Superior (first)	} part of duodenum	
47	Descending (second)		
48	Horizontal (third)		
49	Right	} kidney	
50	Left		
51	Right	} renal vein	
52	Left		
53	Right	} renal artery	
54	Left		
55	Renal pelvis		
56	Ascending colon		
57	Right colic (hepatic) flexure		
58	Transverse colon		
59	Left colic (splenic) flexure		
60	Descending colon		
61	Jejunum		
62	Falciform ligament		
63	Body	} of sternum	
64	Xiphoid process		
65	Serratus anterior muscle		
66	Latissimus dorsi muscle		
67	Erector spinae muscle		
68	Trapezius muscle		
69	Rectus abdominis muscle		
70	External oblique muscle		
71	Internal oblique muscle		
72	Transversus abdominis muscle		
73	Psoas major muscle		
74	Quadratus lumborum muscle		
75	Inferior mesenteric vein		
76	Inferior mesenteric artery		
77	Right	} atrium	
78	Left		
79	Common iliac artery		
80	Common iliac vein		
81	Body of vertebra		
82	Intervertebral disc		
83	Thecal sac		
84	Ilium		
85	Lateral part (ala) of sacrum		
86	Sacro-iliac joint		
87	Gluteus medius muscle		
88	Ureter		
89	Gluteus maximus muscle		
90	Iliotibial tract		
91	Internal iliac artery		
92	Superior gluteal artery		
93	Gonadal artery and vein		
94	Ileum		
95	Renal fascia		
96	Perirenal	} fat	
97	Pararenal		

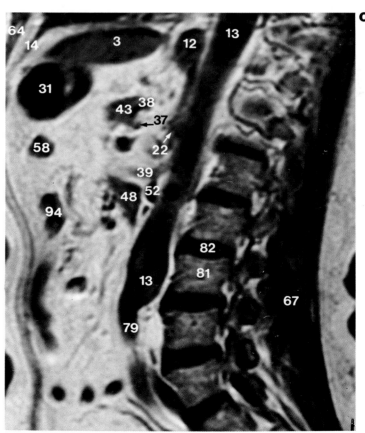

117

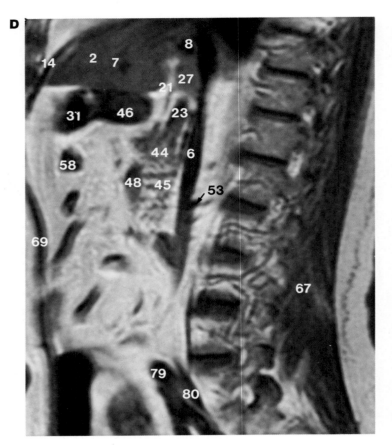

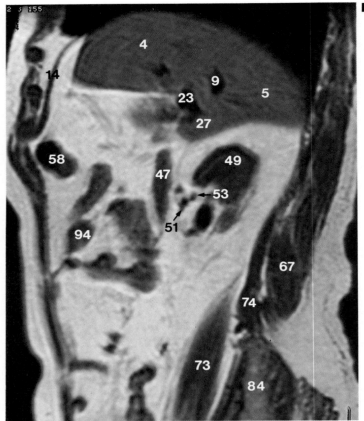

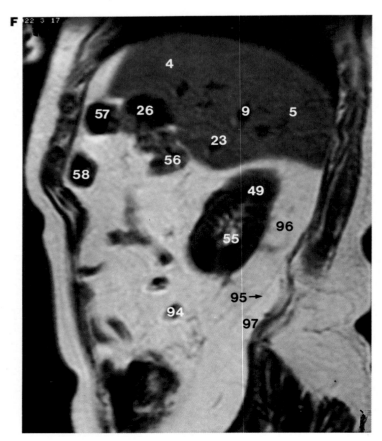

D–F Abdomen. Sagittal MR images (T$_1$-weighted)

1	Right lobe	21	Porta hepatis
2	Medial segment of left lobe	22	Coeliac trunk
3	Lateral segment of left lobe	23	Portal vein
		24	Hepatic artery
4	Anterior segment of right lobe	of liver	25	Common bile duct
		26	Gall bladder
5	Posterior segment of right lobe	27	Caudate lobe of liver
		28	Gastro-oesophageal junction
6	Inferior vena cava	29	Fundus
		30	Body
7	Left		31	Pyloric part	of stomach
8	Middle	hepatic vein	32	Greater curvature
9	Right		33	Lesser curvature
10	Right		34	Left gastric artery
11	Left	ventricle	35	Right	suprarenal gland
12	Oesophagus	36	Left	
13	Aorta	37	Splenic artery
14	Diaphragm	38	Splenic vein
15	Spleen	39	Superior mesenteric artery
16	Azygos vein	40	Superior mesenteric vein
17	Right		41	Tail
18	Left	crus of diaphragm	42	Body	of pancreas
		43	Neck
19	Hemi-azygos vein	44	Head
20	Fissure for ligamentum venosum	45	Uncinate process of head

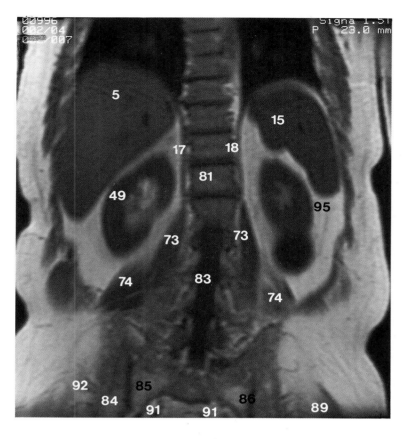

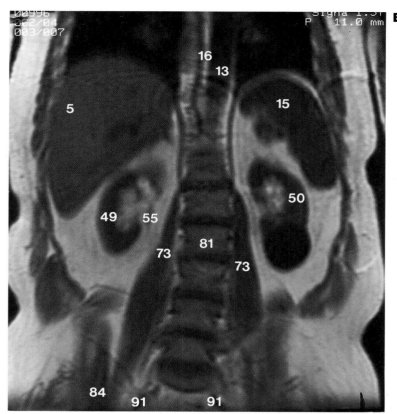

A–F Abdomen. Coronal MR images (T$_1$-weighted)

46	Superior (first)	
47	Descending (second)	part of duodenum
48	Horizontal (third)	
49	Right	kidney
50	Left	
51	Right	renal vein
52	Left	
53	Right	renal artery
54	Left	
55	Renal pelvis	
56	Ascending colon	
57	Right colic (hepatic) flexure	
58	Transverse colon	
59	Left colic (splenic) flexure	
60	Descending colon	
61	Jejunum	
62	Falciform ligament	
63	Body	of sternum
64	Xiphoid process	
65	Serratus anterior muscle	
66	Latissimus dorsi muscle	
67	Erector spinae muscle	
68	Trapezius muscle	
69	Rectus abdominis muscle	
70	External oblique muscle	
71	Internal oblique muscle	
72	Transversus abdominis muscle	
73	Psoas major muscle	
74	Quadratus lumborum muscle	
75	Inferior mesenteric vein	
76	Inferior mesenteric artery	
77	Right	atrium
78	Left	
79	Common iliac artery	
80	Common iliac vein	
81	Body of vertebra	
82	Intervertebral disc	
83	Thecal sac	
84	Ilium	
85	Lateral part (ala) of sacrum	
86	Sacro-iliac joint	
87	Gluteus medius muscle	
88	Ureter	
89	Gluteus maximus muscle	
90	Iliotibial tract	
91	Internal iliac artery	
92	Superior gluteal artery	
93	Gonadal artery and vein	
94	Ileum	
95	Renal fascia	
96	Perirenal	fat
97	Pararenal	

● Note the small left renal cyst.

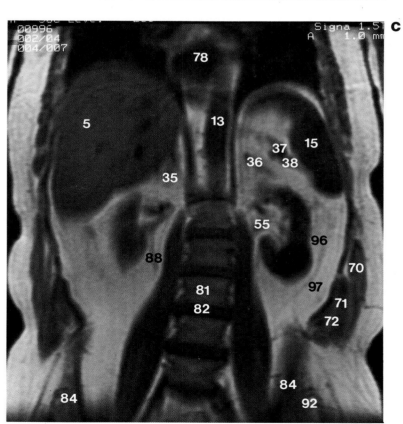

D

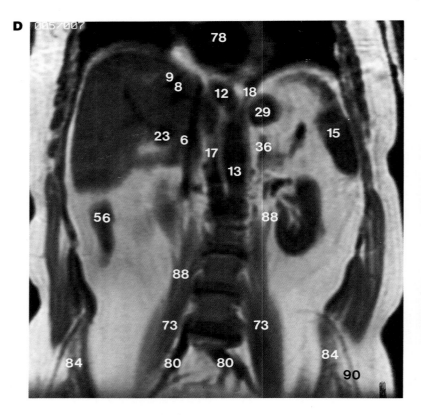

E

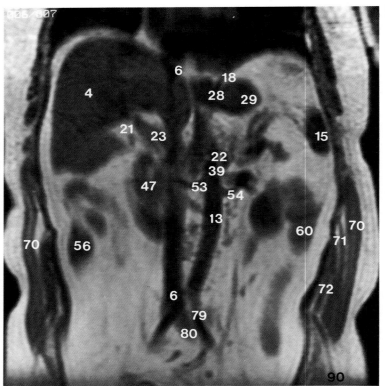

F

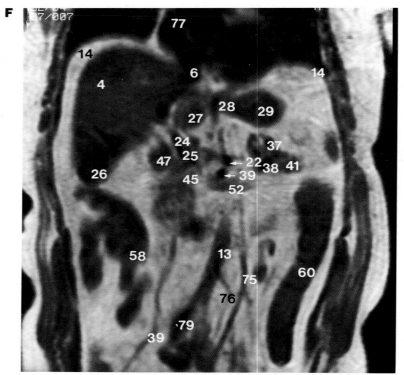

D–F Abdomen. Coronal MR images (T$_1$-weighted)

For Key, see pp. 118–119

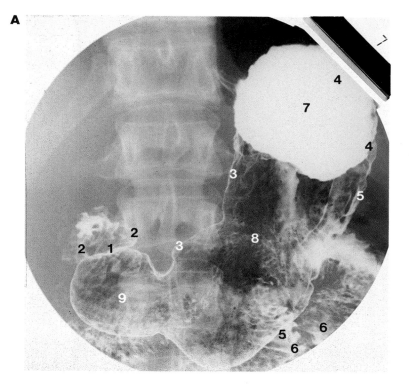

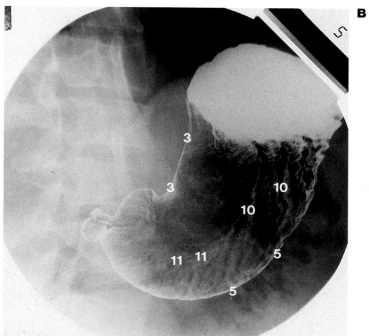

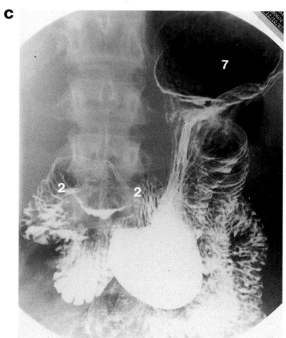

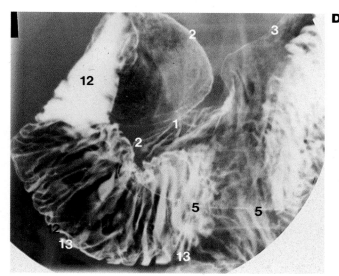

Abdomen. Double-contrast barium meals of stomach and duodenum, **A** and **B** with the patient supine (to show the mucosa of the stomach), **C** with the patient erect, **D** with the patient in a supine oblique position (to show the duodenum)

1	Region of pyloric canal
2	Duodenal cap (superior (first) part of duodenum)
3	Lesser curvature
4	Barium pooling in fundus } of stomach
5	Greater curvature
6	Small bowel
7	Fundus
8	Body } of stomach
9	Antrum
10	Rugae
11	Gas bubbles
12	Descending (second) part } of duodenum
13	Horizontal (third) part

121

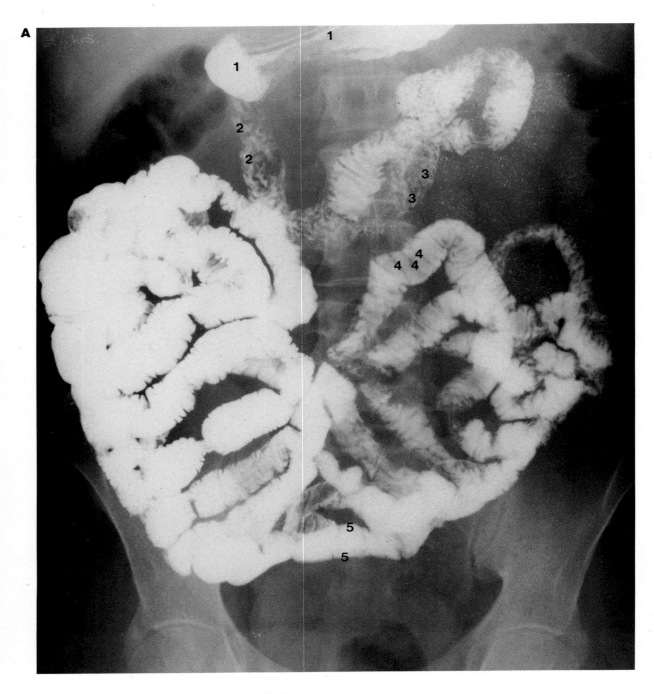

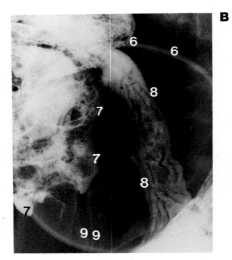

Abdomen. Barium follow-throughs, A with the patient supine, B showing a localised view of the terminal ileum. Anteroposterior radiographs

1 Stomach	6 Compression device
2 Descending (second) part of duodenum	7 Caecum
3 Proximal jejunum	8 Terminal ileum
4 Valvulae conniventes (plicae circulares) of jejunum	9 Right sacro-iliac joint
5 Proximal ileum	

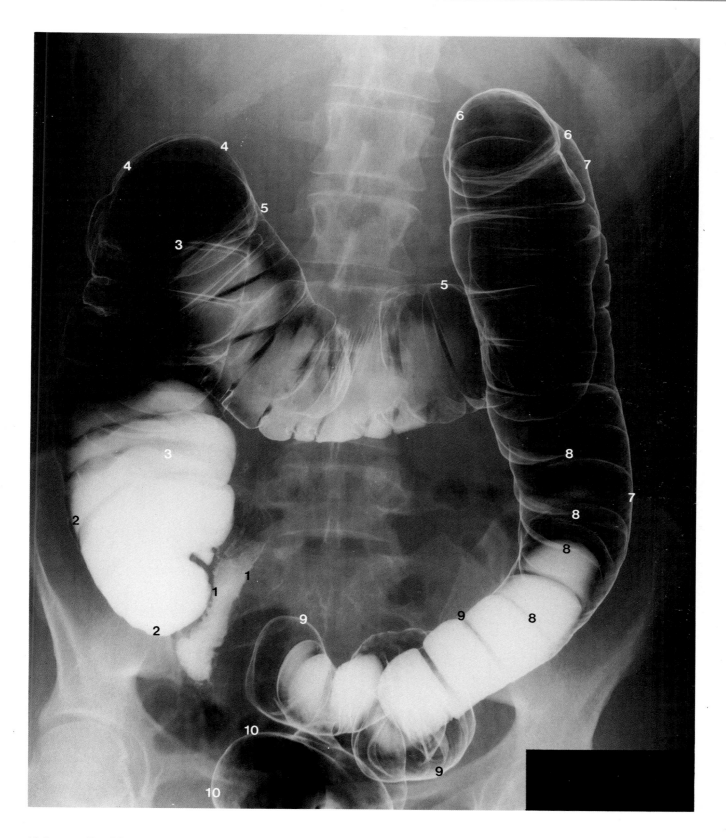

Abdomen. Double-contrast barium enema of the large bowel (colon)

1	Terminal ileum	9	Sigmoid colon
2	Caecum	10	Rectum
3	Ascending portion		
4	Right colic (hepatic) flexure		
5	Transverse portion	of colon	
6	Left colic (splenic) flexure		
7	Descending portion		
8	Sacculations (haustrations)		

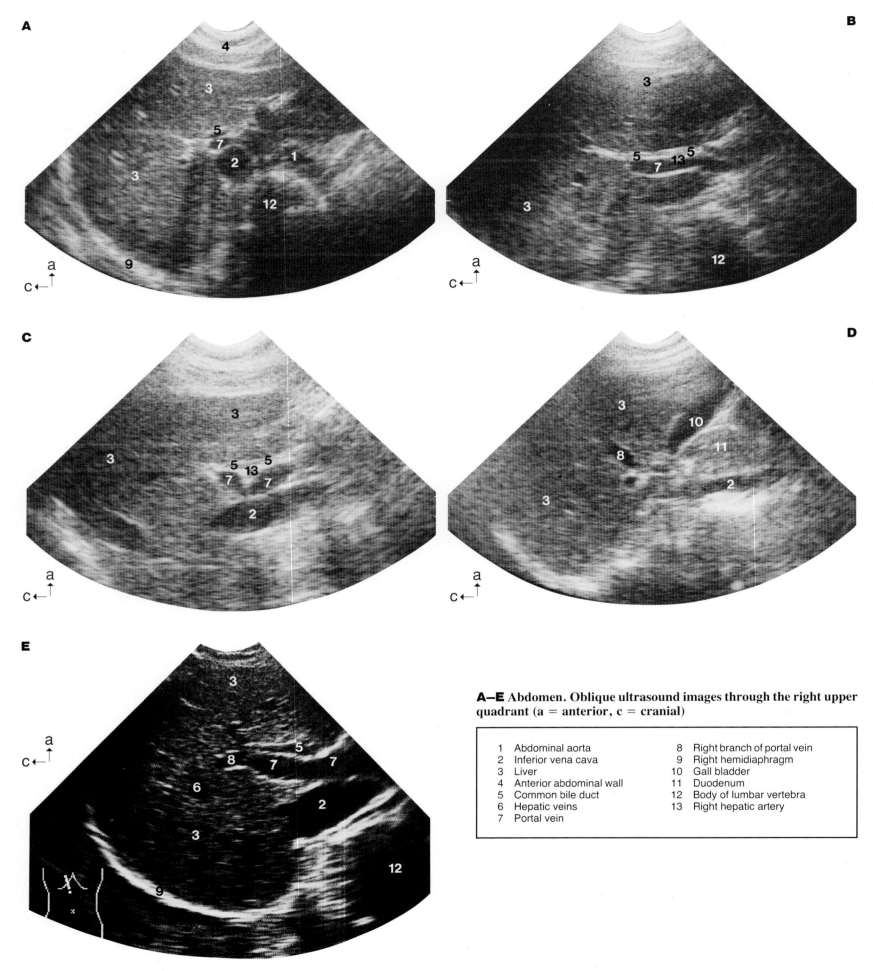

A—E Abdomen. Oblique ultrasound images through the right upper quadrant (a = anterior, c = cranial)

1	Abdominal aorta	8	Right branch of portal vein
2	Inferior vena cava	9	Right hemidiaphragm
3	Liver	10	Gall bladder
4	Anterior abdominal wall	11	Duodenum
5	Common bile duct	12	Body of lumbar vertebra
6	Hepatic veins	13	Right hepatic artery
7	Portal vein		

124

A and **B** Subtracted coeliac trunk
arteriograms

1	Tip of catheter in coeliac trunk
2	Splenic artery
3	Left gastric artery
4	Hepatic artery
5	Gastroduodenal artery
6	Superior pancreaticoduodenal artery
7	Right ⎫ hepatic artery
8	Left ⎭
9	Dorsal pancreatic artery
10	Left ⎫ gastro-epiploic
11	Right ⎭ artery
12	Phrenic artery
13	Transverse pancreatic artery
14	Pancreatica magna artery

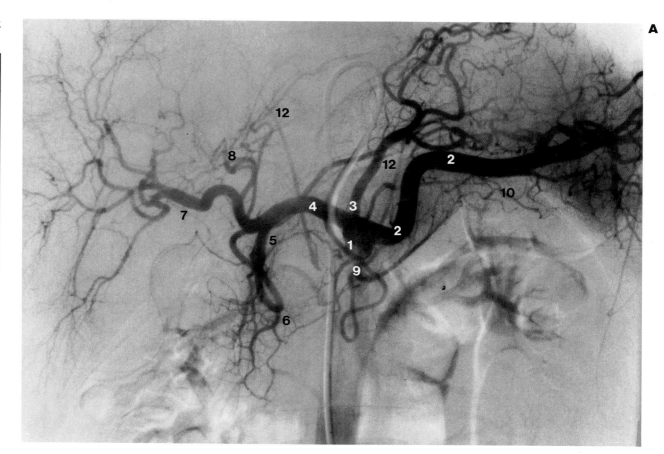

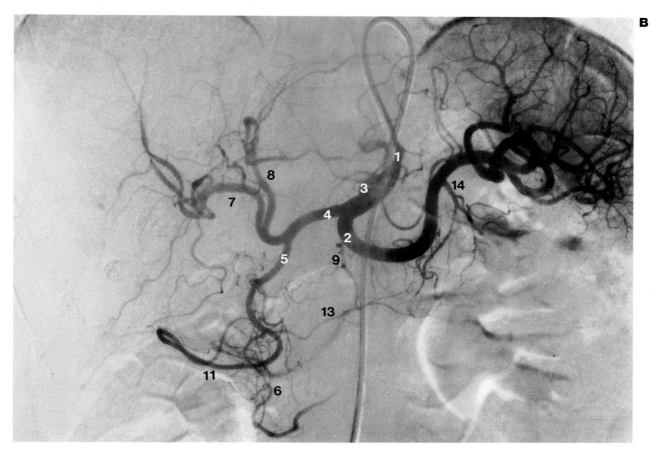

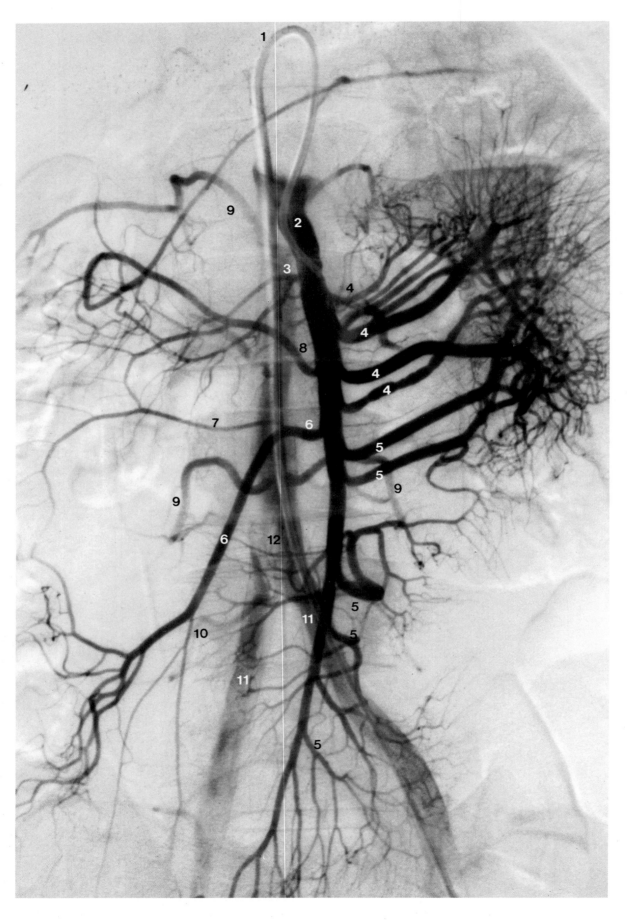

Subtracted superior mesenteric arteriogram

1	Catheter with tip selectively in superior mesenteric artery
2	Superior mesenteric artery
3	Inferior pancreaticoduodenal artery
4	Jejunal branches } of superior
5	Ileal branches } mesenteric artery
6	Ileocolic artery
7	Right colic artery
8	Middle colic artery
9	Lumbar arteries arising from abdominal aorta
10	Appendicular artery
11	Iliac artery
12	Aorta

A

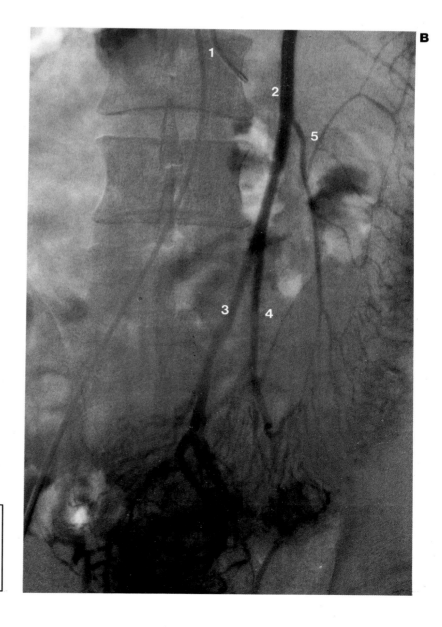

A Subtracted inferior mesenteric arteriogram

1 Tip of catheter in inferior mesenteric artery
2 Inferior mesenteric artery
3 Left colic artery
4 Ascending ⎫
5 Descending ⎬ branch of left colic artery
6 Sigmoid arteries
7 Superior rectal artery

B Venous phase of subtracted inferior mesenteric arteriogram

1 Tip of catheter in inferior mesenteric artery
2 Inferior mesenteric vein
3 Superior rectal vein
4 Sigmoid vein
5 Left colic vein

B

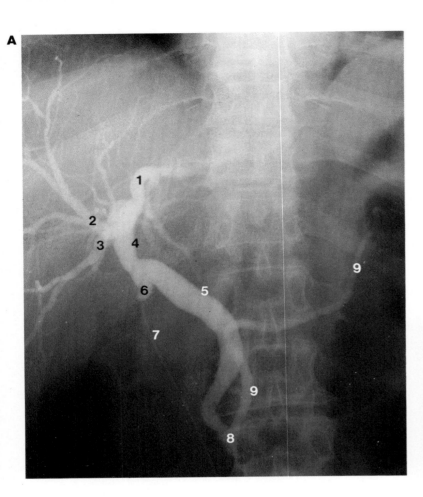

A Peroperative cholangiogram

1	Left hepatic duct
2	Dorsal ⎫
3	Ventral ⎬ branch of right hepatic duct
4	Common hepatic duct
5	Common bile duct
6	Stump of cystic duct
7	Catheter
8	Hepatopancreatic (Vater's) ampulla
9	Pancreatic duct

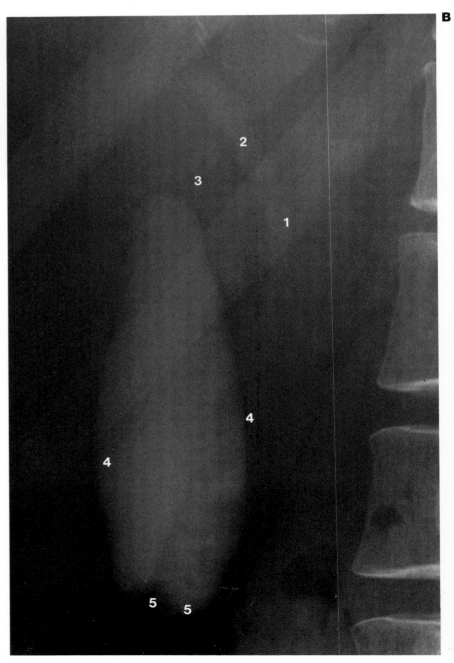

B Oral cholecystogram, with the patient prone. Oblique image

1	Common bile duct
2	Common hepatic duct
3	Cystic duct
4	Body ⎫
5	Fundus ⎬ of gall bladder

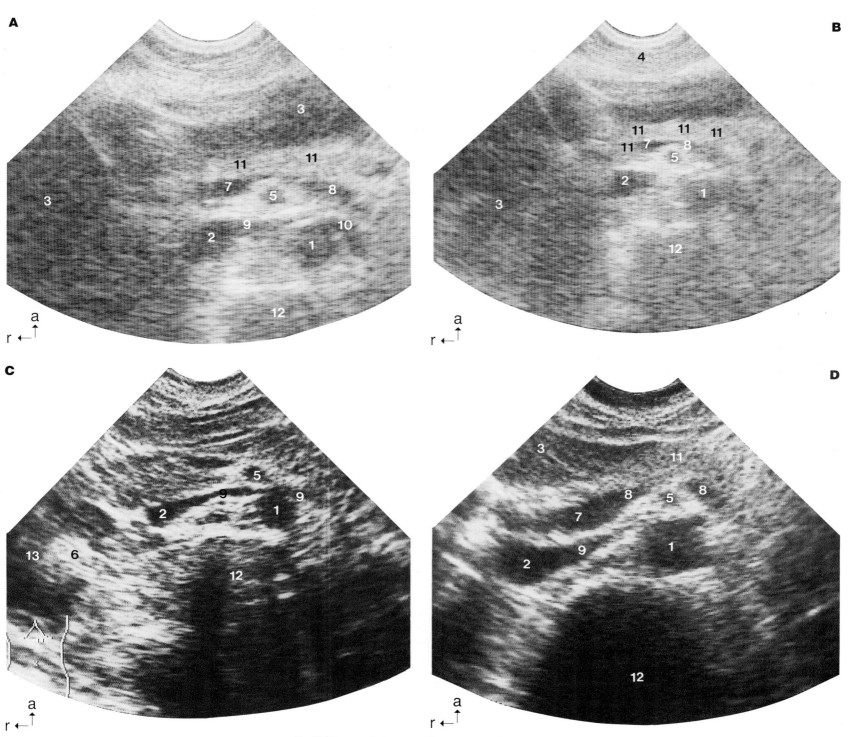

A–D Upper abdomen. Transverse ultrasound images (a = anterior, r = right)

1	Abdominal aorta
2	Inferior vena cava
3	Liver
4	Anterior abdominal wall
5	Superior mesenteric artery
6	Fat in renal sinus
7	Portal vein
8	Splenic vein
9	Left renal vein
10	Left renal artery
11	Pancreas
12	Body of lumbar vertebra
13	Right kidney

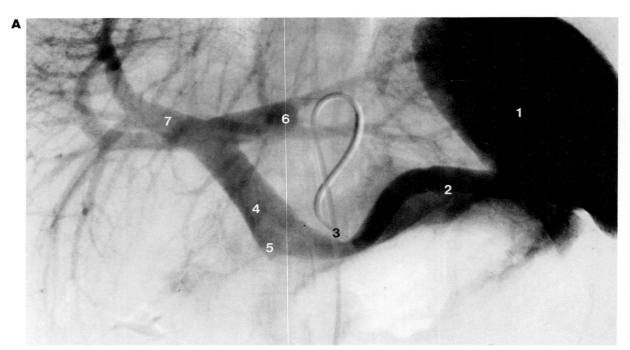

A Indirect splenoportogram

1 Spleen
2 Splenic vein
3 Tip of catheter in splenic artery
4 Portal vein
5 Entry of superior mesenteric vein
6 Left ⎫
7 Right ⎭ branch of portal vein

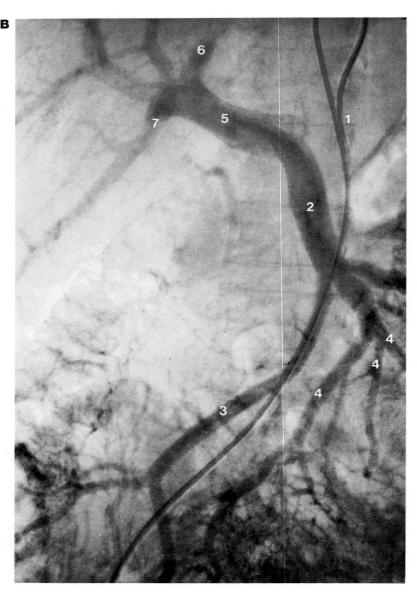

B Venous phase of superior mesenteric arteriogram

1 Tip of catheter in superior mesenteric artery
2 Superior mesenteric vein
3 Ileocolic vein
4 Jejunal vein
5 Portal vein
6 Left ⎫
7 Right ⎭ branch of portal vein

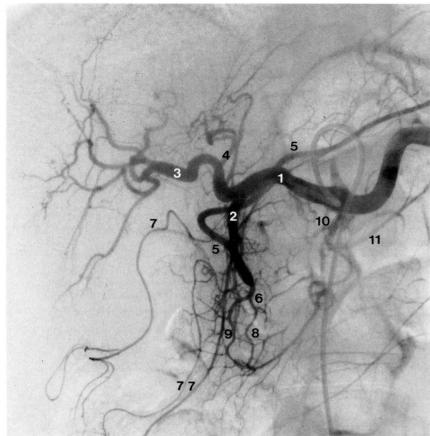

A Subtracted hepatic arteriogram

1	Tip of catheter in hepatic artery
2	Gastroduodenal artery
3	Right ⎫
4	Left ⎭ branch of hepatic artery
5	Right gastro-epiploic artery
6	Superior pancreaticoduodenal artery
7	Epiploic arteries
8	Posterior ⎫ branch of superior
9	Anterior ⎭ pancreaticoduodenal artery
10	Dorsal pancreatic artery
11	Transverse pancreatic artery

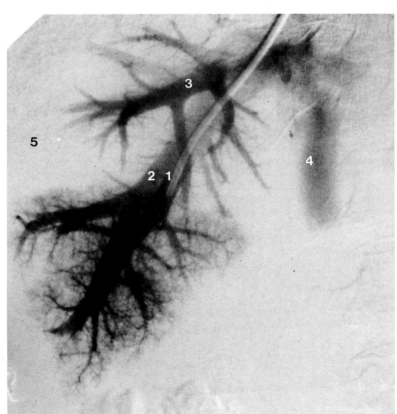

B Subtracted hepatic venogram

1	Tip of catheter in hepatic vein
2	Right ⎫
3	Middle ⎭ hepatic vein
4	Inferior vena cava
5	Parenchyma of liver

131

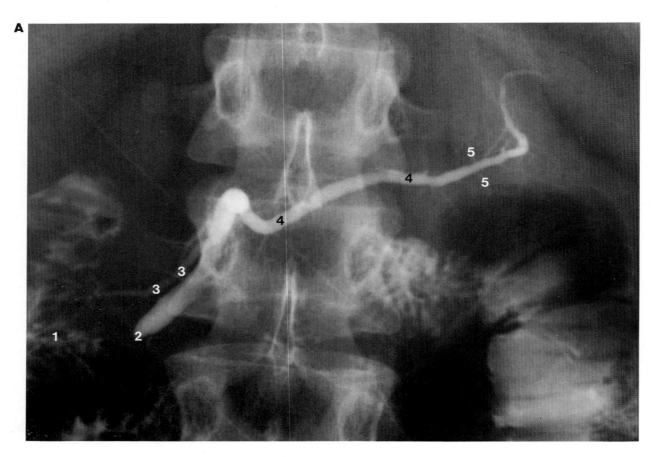

A Endoscopic retrograde cholangiopancreatogram

1	Contrast and gas in descending (second) part of duodenum
2	Ampullary part of pancreatic duct
3	Accessory pancreatic (Santorini's) duct
4	Main pancreatic duct
5	Intralobular ducts

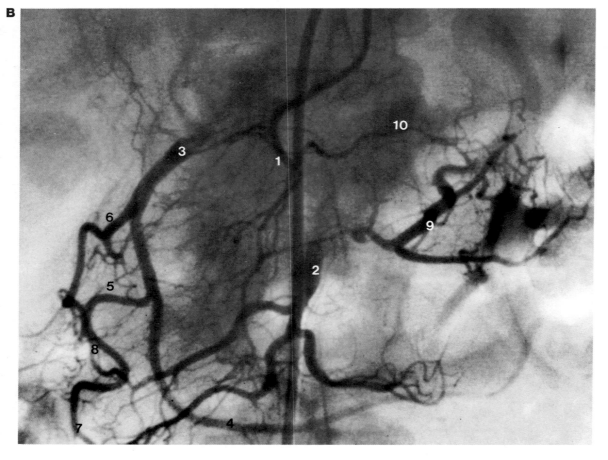

B Subtracted pancreatic arteriogram

1	Tip of catheter in dorsal pancreatic artery
2	Superior mesenteric artery
3	Gastroduodenal artery
4	Right gastro-epiploic artery
5	Anterior ⎱ branch of superior
6	Posterior ⎰ pancreaticoduodenal artery
7	Anterior ⎱ branch of inferior
8	Posterior ⎰ pancreaticoduodenal artery
9	Left gastro-epiploic artery
10	Transverse pancreatic artery

A Nephrographic phase of an excretion urogram

1	Upper pole	} of left kidney
2	Lateral margin	
3	Lower pole	
4	Left psoas muscle	
5	Gas in stomach	
6	Right psoas muscle	
7	Gas in transverse colon	
8	Lower pole	} of right kidney
9	Lateral border	
10	Upper pole	

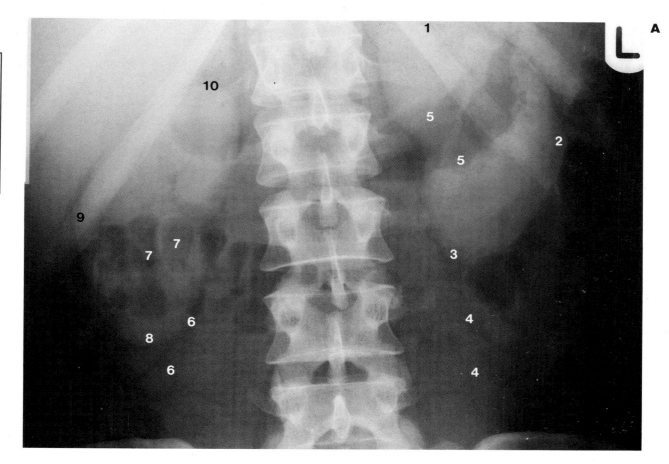

B Pyelographic phase of an excretion urogram (a = upper pole cortex of right kidney, b = central cortex of right kidney, c = lower pole cortex of right kidney)

The interpapillary line, which is indicated by the dotted line, represents the innermost border of the renal cortex.

1	Upper pole of left kidney
2	Renal papilla
3	Minor } calyx
4	Major
5	Renal pelvis
6	Lower pole of left kidney
7	Left ureter

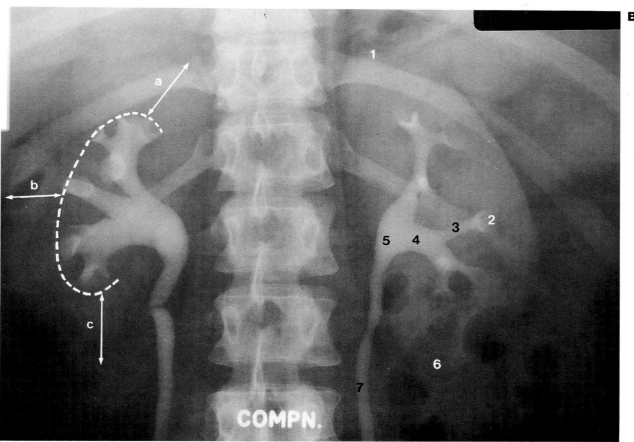

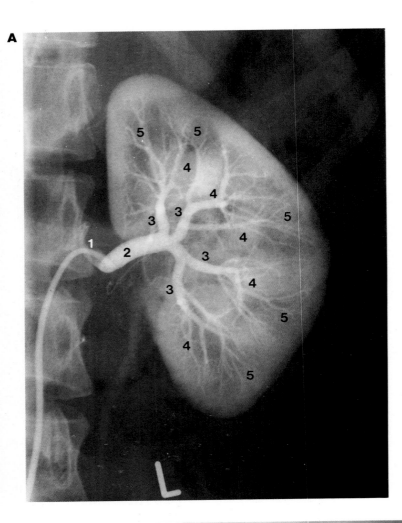

A Renal arteriogram

1	Tip of catheter in renal artery
2	Main renal artery
3	Lobar arteries
4	Interlobar arteries
5	Arcuate arteries

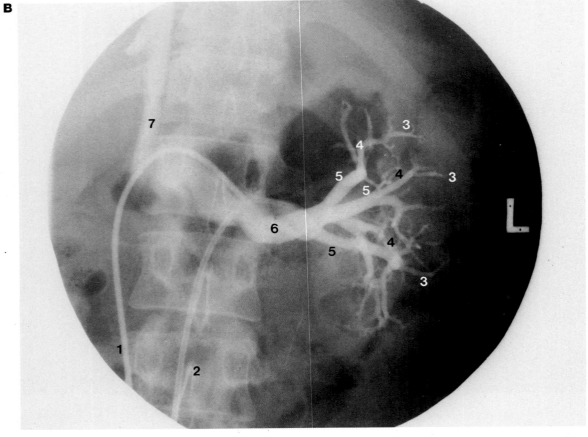

B Left renal venogram

1	Catheter in left renal vein
2	Catheter in left renal artery
3	Arcuate veins
4	Interlobar veins
5	Lobar veins
6	Main renal vein
7	Inferior vena cava

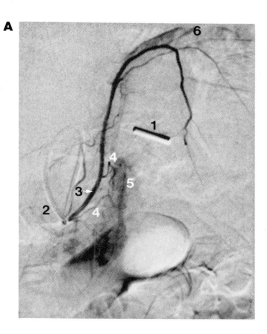

A Left suprarenal arteriogram

1	Tip of nasogastric tube
2	Catheter in origin of inferior phrenic artery
3	Inferior phrenic artery
4	Superior suprarenal arteries
5	Left suprarenal gland
6	Diaphragm

B Left suprarenal venogram

Angiography of the suprarenal glands has been superseded by other imaging techniques. Although there is a wide variation, the arterial supply to the suprarenal glands is from three main arteries: the inferior suprarenal artery, which comes off the renal artery; the middle suprarenal artery, directly off the aorta; and the superior suprarenal artery, arising from the inferior phrenic artery.

Suprarenal venous sampling is still performed in some centres as part of the localisation of hormone-secreting tumours.

1	Tip of catheter in left suprarenal vein
2	Left renal vein
3	Capsular veins
4	Upper pole calyx
5	Adenoma in suprarenal gland
6	Inferior phrenic vein

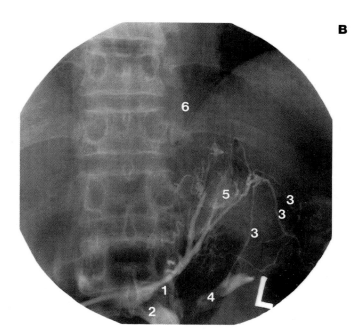

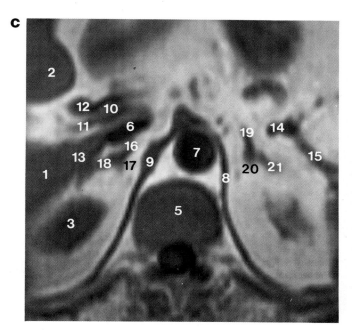

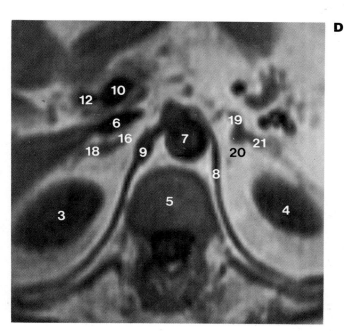

C and D
Suprarenal glands.
Axial MR images
(T₁-weighted)

1	Right	} lobe of liver	
2	Medial segment of left		
3	Right	} kidney	
4	Left		
5	Body of vertebra		
6	Inferior vena cava		
7	Aorta		
8	Left	} crus of diaphragm	
9	Right		
10	Portal vein		
11	Hepatic artery		
12	Common bile duct		
13	Caudate lobe of liver		
14	Splenic artery		
15	Splenic vein		
16	Body	} of right suprarenal gland	
17	Medial limb		
18	Lateral limb		
19	Body	} of left suprarenal gland	
20	Medial limb		
21	Lateral limb		

135

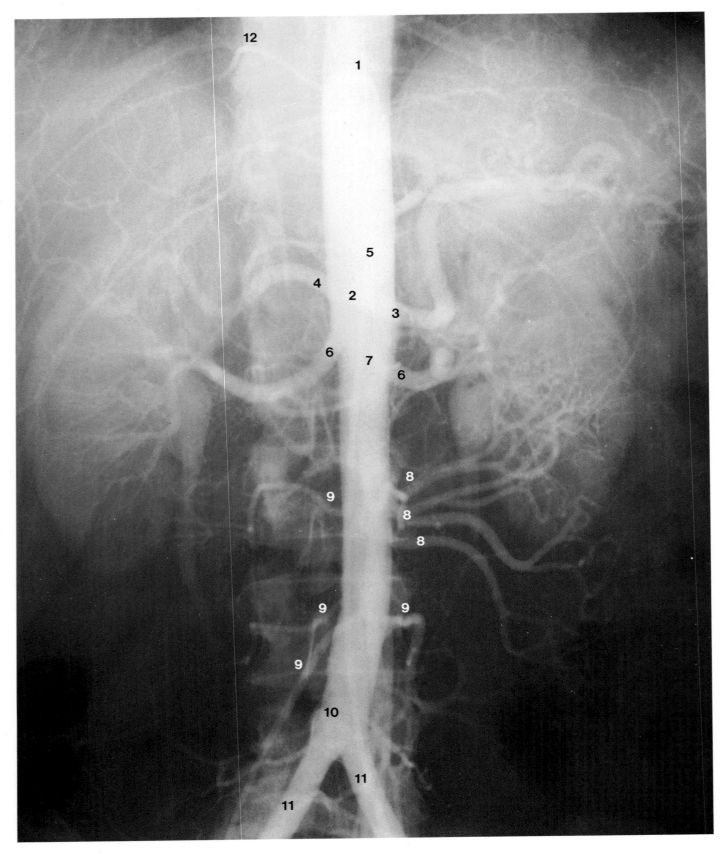

Abdominal aortogram

1	Tip of pigtail catheter in abdominal aorta	5	Left gastric artery	9	Lumbar arteries
2	Coeliac trunk	6	Renal artery	10	Abdominal aorta
3	Splenic artery	7	Superior mesenteric artery	11	Common iliac arteries
4	Hepatic artery	8	Jejunal branches of superior mesenteric artery	12	Intercostal artery

Inferior vena cavogram

1	Inferior vena cava
2	Entrance of hepatic veins
3	Entrance of renal veins
4	Common iliac vein
5	Internal iliac vein
6	External iliac vein
7	Iliolumbar vein
8	Ascending lumbar vein

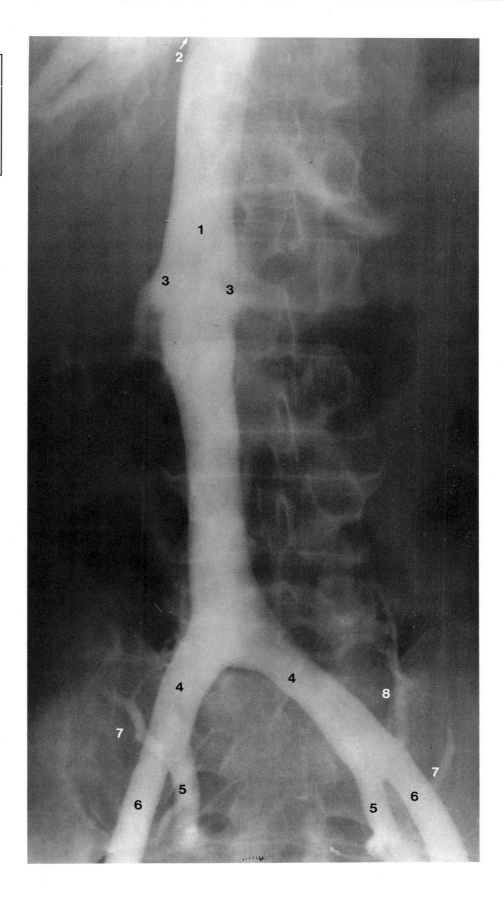

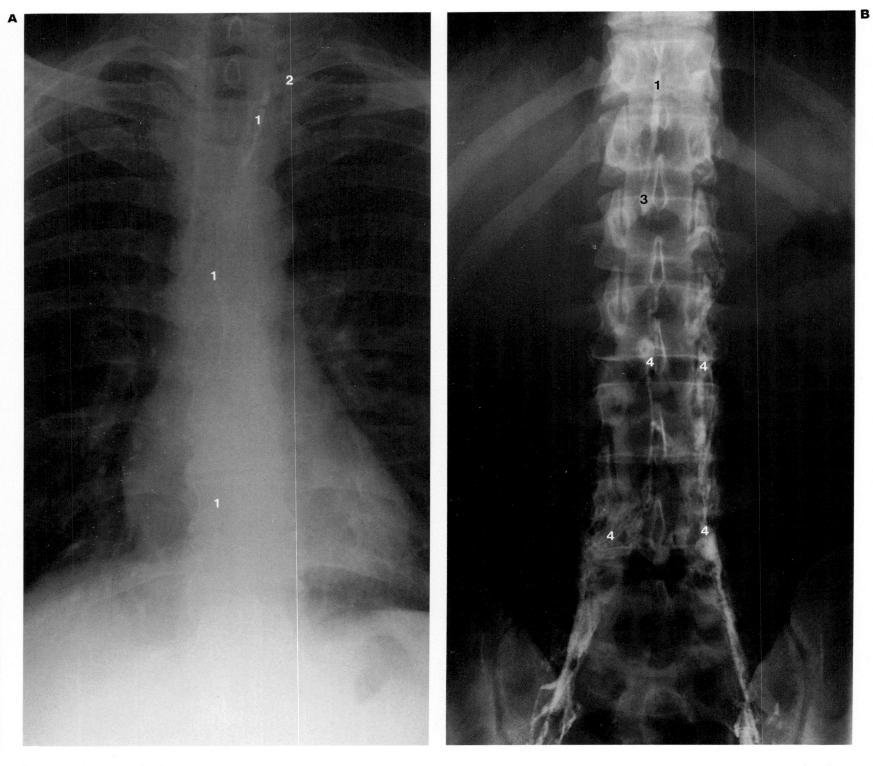

Lymphangiograms, A of the thorax and upper abdomen, B of the paralumbar region, C of the pelvic region

1	Thoracic duct	5	External iliac nodes ⎫
2	Terminal ampulla	6	Inguinal nodes ⎬ (early filling)
3	Cisterna chyli	7	Efferent inguinal lymphatics
4	Ascending lumbar chains		

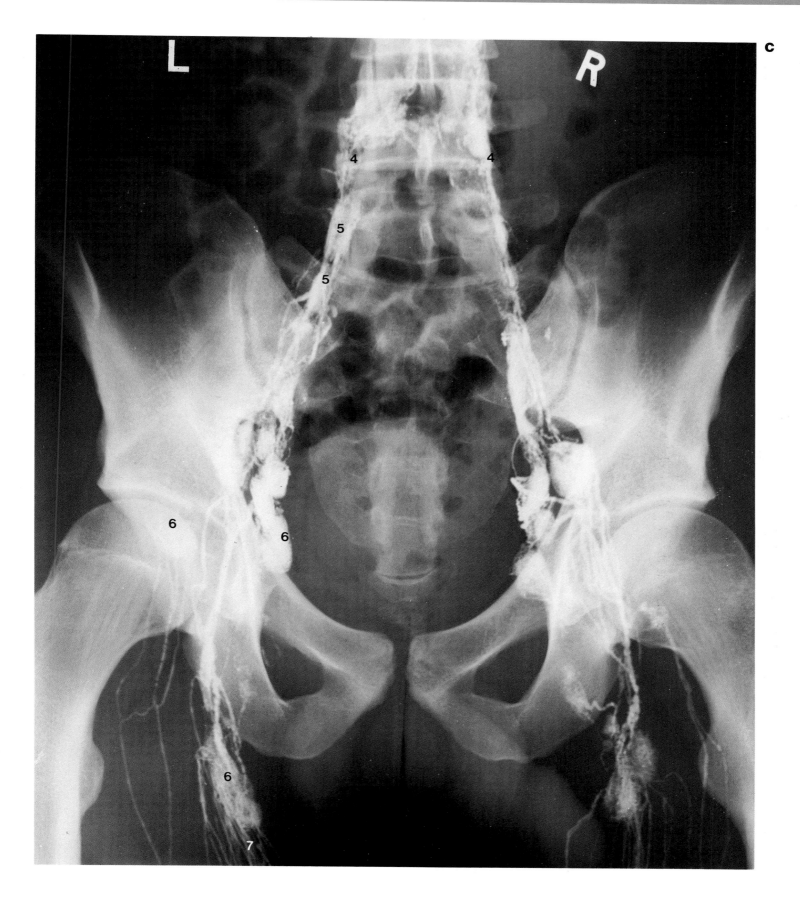

Pelvis

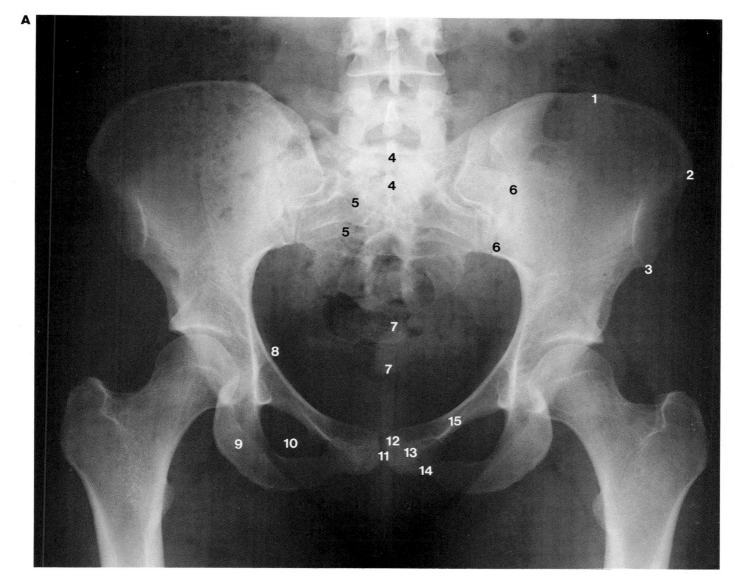

A

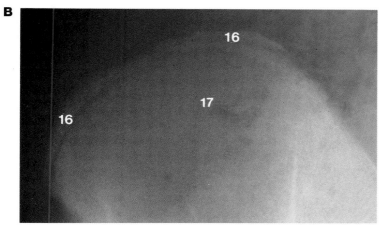

B

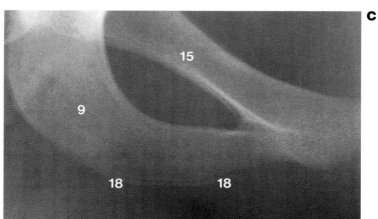

C

A Pelvis and hips of an adult female. Anteroposterior projection

B and **C** Pelvis of a 17-year-old boy. Anteroposterior projections

1	Iliac crest	10	Obturator foramen
2	Anterior superior iliac spine	11	Pubic symphysis
3	Anterior inferior iliac spine	12	Tubercle
4	Sacral crest	13	Body } of pubis
5	Anterior sacral foramen	14	Inferior ramus
6	Sacro-iliac joint	15	Superior ramus
7	Segment of coccyx	16	Centre for iliac crest
8	Ischial spine	17	Ilium
9	Ischial ramus	18	Centre for ischial tuberosity

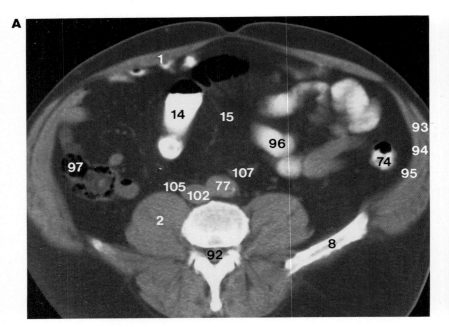

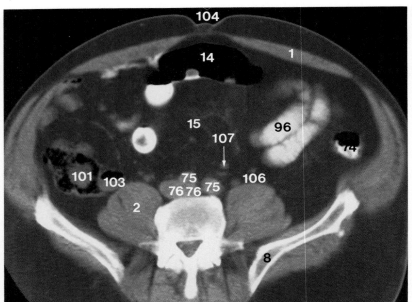

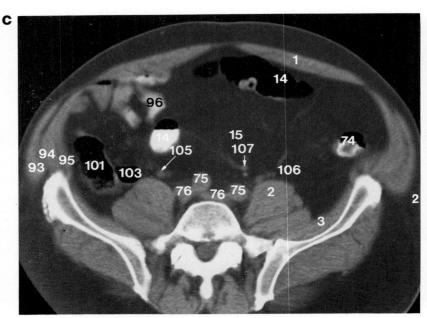

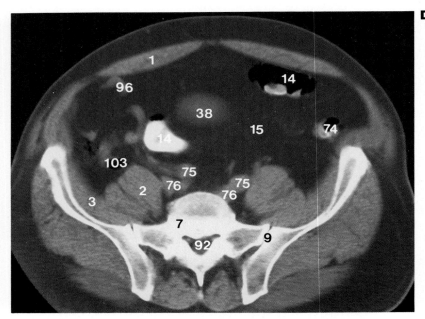

A—H Male pelvis. Axial CT images

1	Rectus abdominis muscle	15	Mesenteric fat	29	Obturator artery and vein	42	Greater trochanter } of femur
2	Psoas muscle	16	Sacral plexus	30	Femoral artery	43	Ligament of head } of femur
3	Iliacus muscle	17	Dorsal } sacral foramen	31	Femoral vein	44	Ischial spine
4	Gluteus minimus muscle	18	Ventral } sacral foramen	32	Inferior gluteal artery and vein	45	Ischium
5	Gluteus medius muscle	19	Piriformis muscle			46	Superior ramus of pubis
6	Gluteus maximus muscle	20	Superior gluteal artery and vein	33	Gemellus muscle	47	Prostate
7	Sacrum	21	Sartorius muscle	34	Rectum	48	Levator ani muscle
8	Ilium	22	Iliotibial tract	35	Acetabular roof	49	Neck of femur
9	Sacroiliac joint	23	Tensor fasciae latae muscle	36	Acetabulum	50	Spermatic cord
10	External iliac artery			37	Head of femur	51	Pectineus muscle
11	External iliac vein	24	Iliopsoas muscle	38	Dome of bladder	52	Prostatic urethra
12	Internal iliac artery	25	Greater sciatic foramen	39	Bladder	53	Obturator externus muscle
13	Internal iliac vein	26	Sciatic nerve	40	Seminal vesicle	54	Vastus lateralis muscle
14	Sigmoid colon	27	Femoral nerve	41	Rectus femoris muscle	55	Sacrotuberous ligament
		28	Obturator internus muscle				

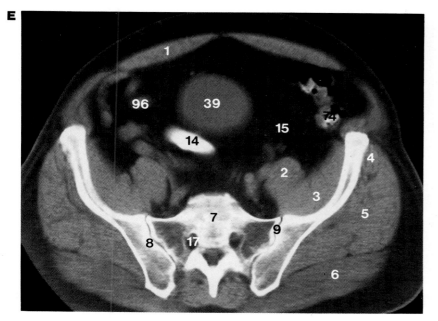

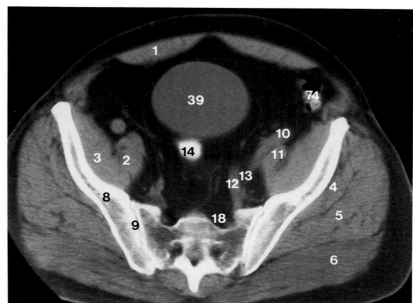

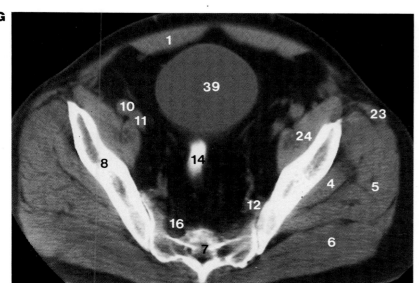

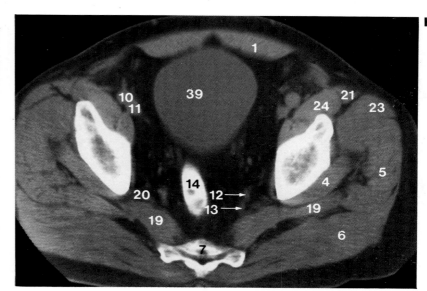

56	Ischioanal fossa	70	Quadratus femoris muscle	84	Semitendinosus muscle	98	External anal sphincter
57	Pubic symphysis	71	Vastus intermedius muscle	85	Semimembranosus muscle	99	Biceps femoris muscle
58	Adductor brevis muscle	72	Superficial femoral artery	86	Gracilis muscle	100	Lesser trochanter of femur
59	Adductor longus muscle	73	Profunda femoris artery	87	Ejaculatory duct	101	Caecum
60	Anal canal	74	Descending colon	88	Body of pubis	102	Inferior vena cava
61	Membranous urethra	75	Common iliac artery	89	Testis	103	Terminal ileum
62	Inferior ramus of pubis	76	Common iliac artery/vein	90	Epididymis	104	Umbilicus
63	Ischial tuberosity	77	Aorta	91	Median sacral artery	105	Ureter
64	Internal pudendal artery and vein	78	Sacrospinous ligament	92	Thecal sac	106	Gonadal artery and vein
65	Corpus cavernosum	79	Lateral part (ala) of sacrum	93	External oblique muscle	107	Inferior mesenteric artery
66	Crus of corpus cavernosum	80	Lumbosacral disc	94	Internal oblique muscle	108	Corpus spongiosum
67	Bulb of penis	81	First sacral segment	95	Transversus abdominis muscle	109	Branches of superior mesenteric artery
68	Great (long) saphenous vein	82	Fifth lumbar vertebra	96	Ileal loop		
69	Adductor magnus muscle	83	Coccyx	97	Ascending colon		

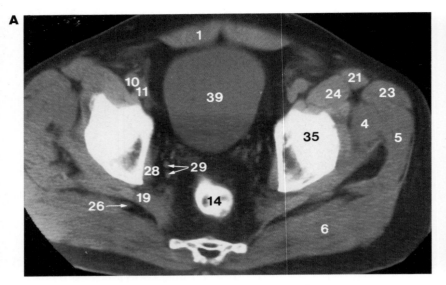
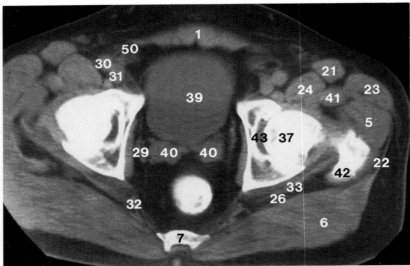
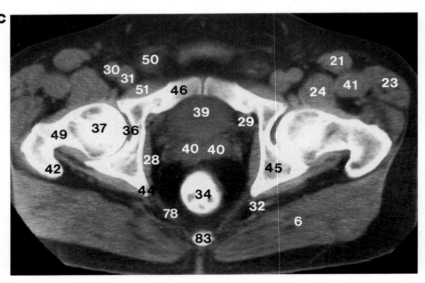
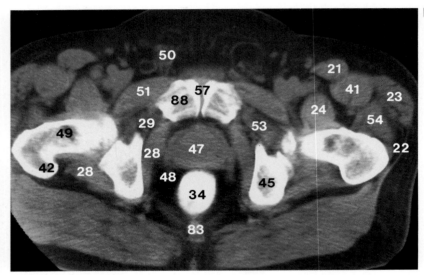

A–I Male pelvis. Axial CT images

1	Rectus abdominis muscle	20	Superior gluteal artery and vein	39	Bladder	58	Adductor brevis muscle
2	Psoas muscle	21	Sartorius muscle	40	Seminal vesicle	59	Adductor longus muscle
3	Iliacus muscle	22	Iliotibial tract	41	Rectus femoris muscle	60	Anal canal
4	Gluteus minimus muscle	23	Tensor fasciae latae muscle	42	Greater trochanter } of femur	61	Membranous urethra
5	Gluteus medius muscle	24	Iliopsoas muscle	43	Ligament of head } of femur	62	Inferior ramus of pubis
6	Gluteus maximus muscle	25	Greater sciatic foramen	44	Ischial spine	63	Ischial tuberosity
7	Sacrum	26	Sciatic nerve	45	Ischium	64	Internal pudendal artery and vein
8	Ilium	27	Femoral nerve	46	Superior ramus of pubis	65	Corpus cavernosum
9	Sacroiliac joint	28	Obturator internus muscle	47	Prostate	66	Crus of corpus cavernosum
10	External iliac artery	29	Obturator artery and vein	48	Levator ani muscle	67	Bulb of penis
11	External iliac vein	30	Femoral artery	49	Neck of femur	68	Great (long) saphenous vein
12	Internal iliac artery	31	Femoral vein	50	Spermatic cord	69	Adductor magnus muscle
13	Internal iliac vein	32	Inferior gluteal artery and vein	51	Pectineus muscle	70	Quadratus femoris muscle
14	Sigmoid colon	33	Gemellus muscle	52	Prostatic urethra	71	Vastus intermedius muscle
15	Mesenteric fat	34	Rectum	53	Obturator externus muscle	72	Superficial femoral artery
16	Sacral plexus	35	Acetabular roof	54	Vastus lateralis muscle	73	Profunda femoris artery
17	Dorsal } sacral foramen	36	Acetabulum	55	Sacrotuberous ligament	74	Descending colon
18	Ventral } sacral foramen	37	Head of femur	56	Ischioanal fossa	75	Common iliac artery
19	Piriformis muscle	38	Dome of bladder	57	Pubic symphysis	76	Common iliac artery/vein

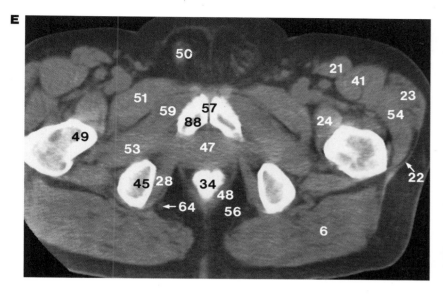

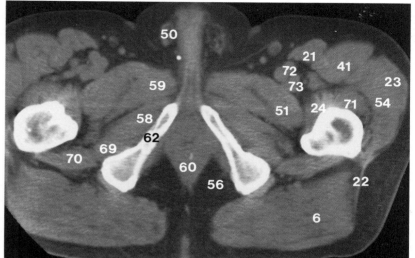

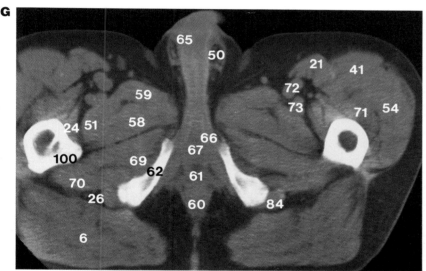

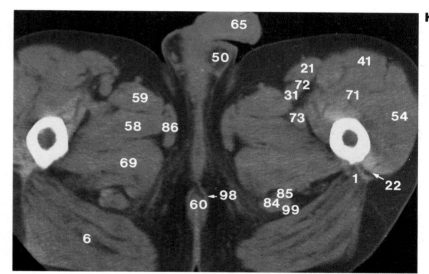

77	Aorta	
78	Sacrospinous ligament	
79	Lateral part (ala) of sacrum	
80	Lumbosacral disc	
81	First sacral segment	
82	Fifth lumbar vertebra	
83	Coccyx	
84	Semitendinosus muscle	
85	Semimembranosus muscle	
86	Gracilis muscle	
87	Ejaculatory duct	
88	Body of pubis	
89	Testis	
90	Epididymis	
91	Median sacral artery	
92	Thecal sac	
93	External oblique muscle	
94	Internal oblique muscle	
95	Transversus abdominis muscle	

96	Ileal loop
97	Ascending colon
98	External anal sphincter
99	Biceps femoris muscle
100	Lesser trochanter of femur
101	Caecum
102	Inferior vena cava
103	Terminal ileum
104	Umbilicus
105	Ureter
106	Gonadal artery and vein
107	Inferior mesenteric artery
108	Corpus spongiosum
109	Branches of superior mesenteric artery

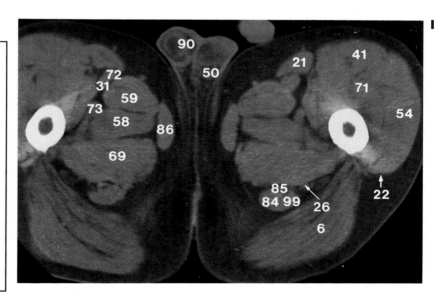

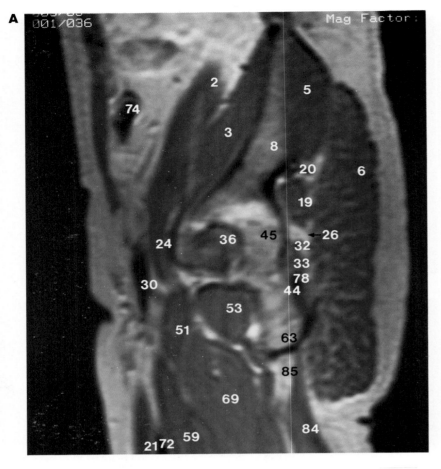

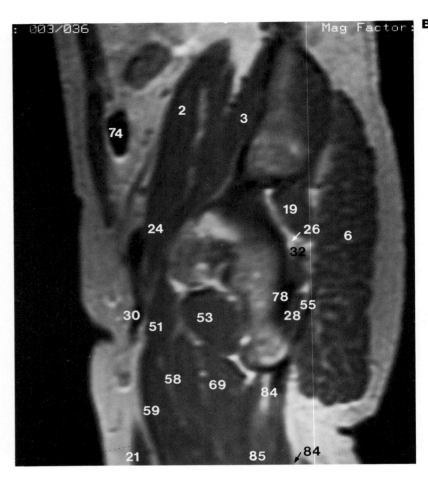

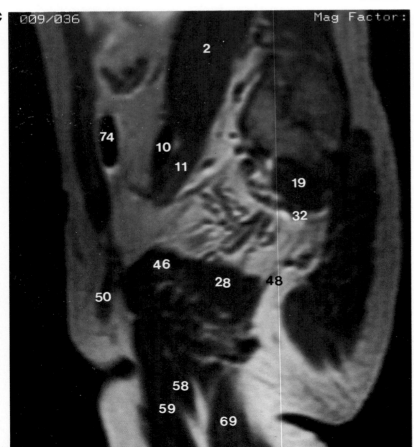

A–F Male pelvis. Sagittal MR images (T₁-weighted)

1	Rectus abdominis muscle	28	Obturator internus muscle
2	Psoas muscle	29	Obturator artery and vein
3	Iliacus muscle	30	Femoral artery
4	Gluteus minimus muscle	31	Femoral vein
5	Gluteus medius muscle	32	Inferior gluteal artery and vein
6	Gluteus maximus muscle	33	Gemellus muscle
7	Sacrum	34	Rectum
8	Ilium	35	Acetabular roof
9	Sacroiliac joint	36	Acetabulum
10	External iliac artery	37	Head of femur
11	External iliac vein	38	Dome of bladder
12	Internal iliac artery	39	Bladder
13	Internal iliac vein	40	Seminal vesicle
14	Sigmoid colon	41	Rectus femoris muscle
15	Mesenteric fat	42	Greater trochanter } of femur
16	Sacral plexus	43	Ligament of head } of femur
17	Dorsal } sacral foramen	44	Ischial spine
18	Ventral } sacral foramen	45	Ischium
19	Piriformis muscle	46	Superior ramus of pubis
20	Superior gluteal artery and vein	47	Prostate
21	Sartorius muscle	48	Levator ani muscle
22	Iliotibial tract	49	Neck of femur
23	Tensor fasciae latae muscle	50	Spermatic cord
24	Iliopsoas muscle	51	Pectineus muscle
25	Greater sciatic foramen	52	Prostatic urethra
26	Sciatic nerve	53	Obturator externus muscle
27	Femoral nerve	54	Vastus lateralis muscle
		55	Sacrotuberous ligament

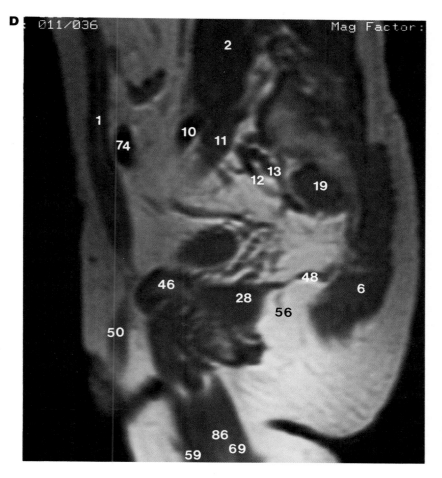

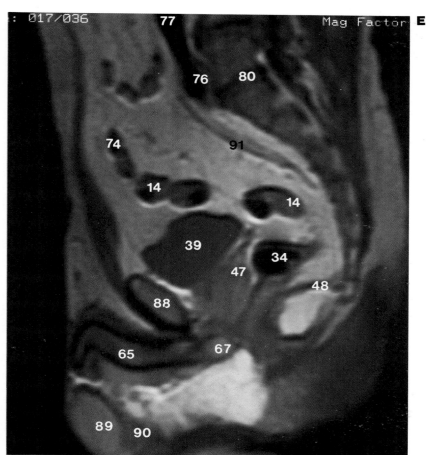

56	Ischioanal fossa	83	Coccyx
57	Pubic symphysis	84	Semitendinosus muscle
58	Adductor brevis muscle	85	Semimembranosus muscle
59	Adductor longus muscle	86	Gracilis muscle
60	Anal canal	87	Ejaculatory duct
61	Membranous urethra	88	Body of pubis
62	Inferior ramus of pubis	89	Testis
63	Ischial tuberosity	90	Epididymis
64	Internal pudendal artery and vein	91	Median sacral artery
65	Corpus cavernosum	92	Thecal sac
66	Crus of corpus cavernosum	93	External oblique muscle
67	Bulb of penis	94	Internal oblique muscle
68	Great (long) saphenous vein	95	Transversus abdominis muscle
69	Adductor magnus muscle	96	Ileal loop
70	Quadratus femoris muscle	97	Ascending colon
71	Vastus intermedius muscle	98	External anal sphincter
72	Superficial femoral artery	99	Biceps femoris muscle
73	Profunda femoris artery	100	Lesser trochanter of femur
74	Descending colon	101	Caecum
75	Common iliac artery	102	Inferior vena cava
76	Common iliac artery/vein	103	Terminal ileum
77	Aorta	104	Umbilicus
78	Sacrospinous ligament	105	Ureter
79	Lateral part (ala) of sacrum	106	Gonadal artery and vein
80	Lumbosacral disc	107	Inferior mesenteric artery
81	First sacral segment	108	Corpus spongiosum
82	Fifth lumbar vertebra	109	Branches of superior mesenteric artery

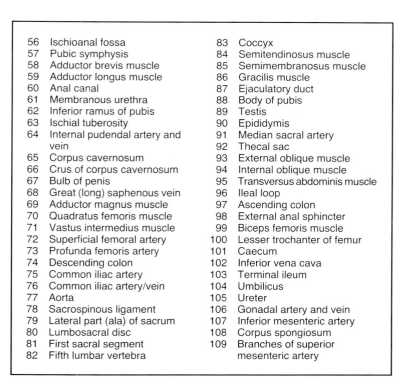

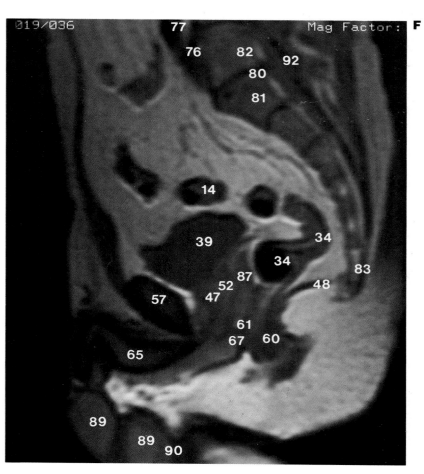

147

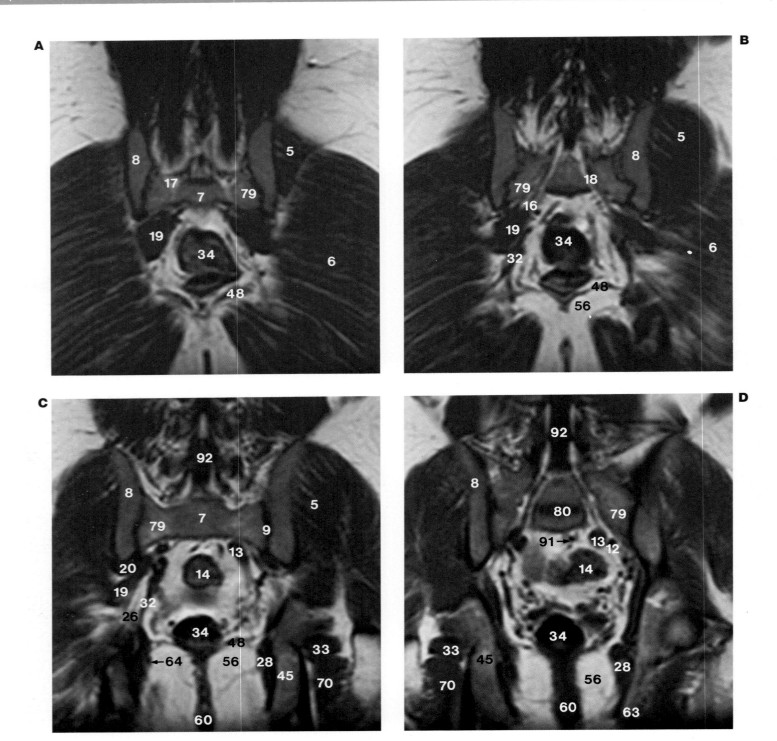

A–H Male pelvis. Coronal MR images (T$_1$-weighted)

1	Rectus abdominis muscle	14	Sigmoid colon	27	Femoral nerve	40	Seminal vesicle
2	Psoas muscle	15	Mesenteric fat	28	Obturator internus muscle	41	Rectus femoris muscle
3	Iliacus muscle	16	Sacral plexus	29	Obturator artery and vein	42	Greater trochanter } of femur
4	Gluteus minimus muscle	17	Dorsal } sacral foramen	30	Femoral artery	43	Ligament of head } of femur
5	Gluteus medius muscle	18	Ventral } sacral foramen	31	Femoral vein	44	Ischial spine
6	Gluteus maximus muscle	19	Piriformis muscle	32	Inferior gluteal artery and vein	45	Ischium
7	Sacrum	20	Superior gluteal artery and vein	33	Gemellus muscle	46	Superior ramus of pubis
8	Ilium	21	Sartorius muscle	34	Rectum	47	Prostate
9	Sacroiliac joint	22	Iliotibial tract	35	Acetabular roof	48	Levator ani muscle
10	External iliac artery	23	Tensor fasciae latae muscle	36	Acetabulum	49	Neck of femur
11	External iliac vein	24	Iliopsoas muscle	37	Head of femur	50	Spermatic cord
12	Internal iliac artery	25	Greater sciatic foramen	38	Dome of bladder	51	Pectineus muscle
13	Internal iliac vein	26	Sciatic nerve	39	Bladder	52	Prostatic urethra

E
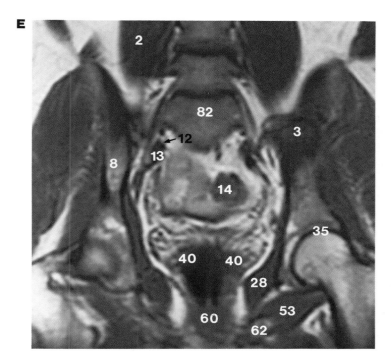

F
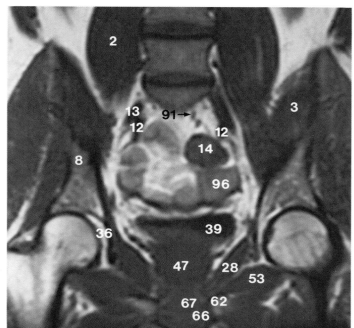

G
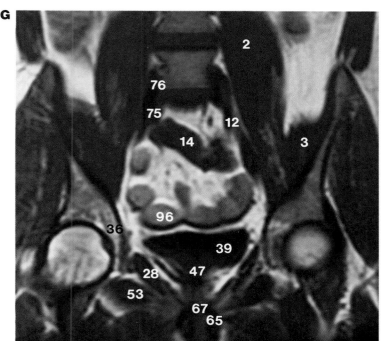

H
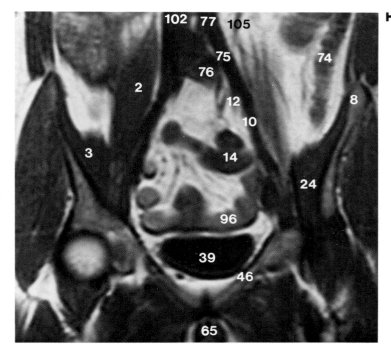

53	Obturator externus muscle	67	Bulb of penis
54	Vastus lateralis muscle	68	Great (long) saphenous vein
55	Sacrotuberous ligament	69	Adductor magnus muscle
56	Ischioanal fossa	70	Quadratus femoris muscle
57	Pubic symphysis	71	Vastus intermedius muscle
58	Adductor brevis muscle	72	Superficial femoral artery
59	Adductor longus muscle	73	Profunda femoris artery
60	Anal canal	74	Descending colon
61	Membranous urethra	75	Common iliac artery
62	Inferior ramus of pubis	76	Common iliac artery/vein
63	Ischial tuberosity	77	Aorta
64	Internal pudendal artery and vein	78	Sacrospinous ligament
65	Corpus cavernosum	79	Lateral part (ala) of sacrum
66	Crus of corpus cavernosum	80	Lumbosacral disc
		81	First sacral segment

82	Fifth lumbar vertebra	96	Ileal loop
83	Coccyx	97	Ascending colon
84	Semitendinosus muscle	98	External anal sphincter
85	Semimembranosus muscle	99	Biceps femoris muscle
86	Gracilis muscle	100	Lesser trochanter of femur
87	Ejaculatory duct	101	Caecum
88	Body of pubis	102	Inferior vena cava
89	Testis	103	Terminal ileum
90	Epididymis	104	Umbilicus
91	Median sacral artery	105	Ureter
92	Thecal sac	106	Gonadal artery and vein
93	External oblique muscle	107	Inferior mesenteric artery
94	Internal oblique muscle	108	Corpus spongiosum
95	Transversus abdominis muscle	109	Branches of superior mesenteric artery

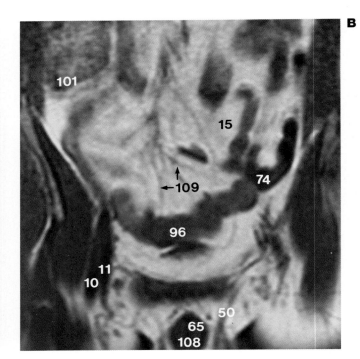

A–C Male pelvis. Coronal MR images (T₁-weighted)

1	Rectus abdominis muscle	42	Greater trochanter } of femur	
2	Psoas muscle	43	Ligament of head } of femur	
3	Iliacus muscle	44	Ischial spine	
4	Gluteus minimus muscle	45	Ischium	
5	Gluteus medius muscle	46	Superior ramus of pubis	
6	Gluteus maximus muscle	47	Prostate	
7	Sacrum	48	Levator ani muscle	
8	Ilium	49	Neck of femur	
9	Sacroiliac joint	50	Spermatic cord	
10	External iliac artery	51	Pectineus muscle	
11	External iliac vein	52	Prostatic urethra	
12	Internal iliac artery	53	Obturator externus muscle	
13	Internal iliac vein	54	Vastus lateralis muscle	
14	Sigmoid colon	55	Sacrotuberous ligament	
15	Mesenteric fat	56	Ischioanal fossa	
16	Sacral plexus	57	Pubic symphysis	
17	Dorsal } sacral foramen	58	Adductor brevis muscle	
18	Ventral } sacral foramen	59	Adductor longus muscle	
19	Piriformis muscle	60	Anal canal	
20	Superior gluteal artery and vein	61	Membranous urethra	
21	Sartorius muscle	62	Inferior ramus of pubis	
22	Iliotibial tract	63	Ischial tuberosity	
23	Tensor fasciae latae muscle	64	Internal pudendal artery and vein	
24	Iliopsoas muscle	65	Corpus cavernosum	
25	Greater sciatic foramen	66	Crus of corpus cavernosum	
26	Sciatic nerve	67	Bulb of penis	
27	Femoral nerve	68	Great (long) saphenous vein	
28	Obturator internus muscle	69	Adductor magnus muscle	
29	Obturator artery and vein	70	Quadratus femoris muscle	
30	Femoral artery	71	Vastus intermedius muscle	
31	Femoral vein	72	Superficial femoral artery	
32	Inferior gluteal artery and vein	73	Profunda femoris artery	
33	Gemellus muscle	74	Descending colon	
34	Rectum	75	Common iliac artery	
35	Acetabular roof	76	Common iliac artery/vein	
36	Acetabulum	77	Aorta	
37	Head of femur	78	Sacrospinous ligament	
38	Dome of bladder	79	Lateral part (ala) of sacrum	
39	Bladder	80	Lumbosacral disc	
40	Seminal vesicle	81	First sacral segment	
41	Rectus femoris muscle	82	Fifth lumbar vertebra	

83	Coccyx	97	Ascending colon
84	Semitendinosus muscle	98	External anal sphincter
85	Semimembranosus muscle	99	Biceps femoris muscle
86	Gracilis muscle	100	Lesser trochanter of femur
87	Ejaculatory duct	101	Caecum
88	Body of pubis	102	Inferior vena cava
89	Testis	103	Terminal ileum
90	Epididymis	104	Umbilicus
91	Median sacral artery	105	Ureter
92	Thecal sac	106	Gonadal artery and vein
93	External oblique muscle	107	Inferior mesenteric artery
94	Internal oblique muscle	108	Corpus spongiosum
95	Transversus abdominis muscle	109	Branches of superior mesenteric artery
96	Ileal loop		

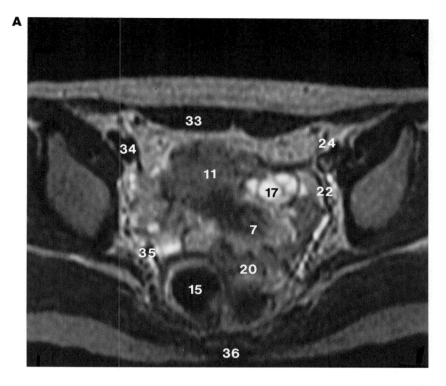

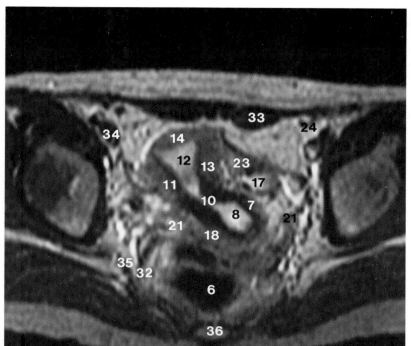

A–C Female pelvis. Axial MR images (T$_2$-weighted)

1	Urethra	22	Ovarian artery
2	Vagina	23	Broad ligament
3	Anterior	24	Round ligament
4	Posterior } fornix of vagina	25	Body of pubis
5	Lateral	26	Pubic symphysis
6	Rectum	27	Obturator internus muscle
7	Wall	28	Ischio-anal fossa
8	Endocervical canal } of cervix	29	Levator ani muscle
9	External os	30	Coccyx
10	Internal os	31	Sacrospinous ligament
11	Myometrium	32	Uterosacral ligament
12	Cavity } of uterus	33	Rectus abdominis muscle
13	Body	34	External iliac artery and vein
14	Fundus	35	Internal iliac artery and vein
15	Sigmoid colon	36	Sacrum
16	Bladder	37	Thecal sac
17	Ovary	38	Vestibule of vagina
18	Recto-uterine pouch	39	Labium majus
19	Anal canal	40	Clitoris
20	Ileum	41	Vesico-uterine pouch
21	Uterine artery		

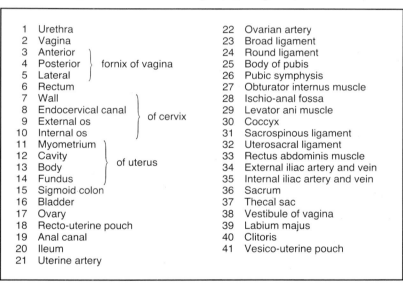

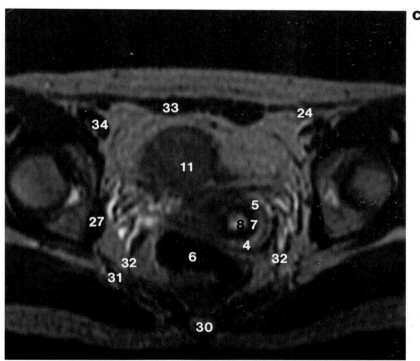

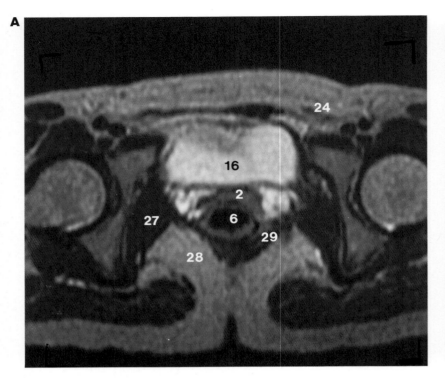

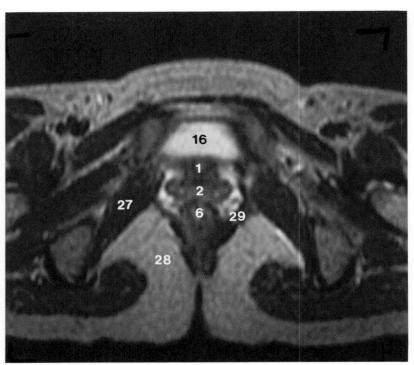

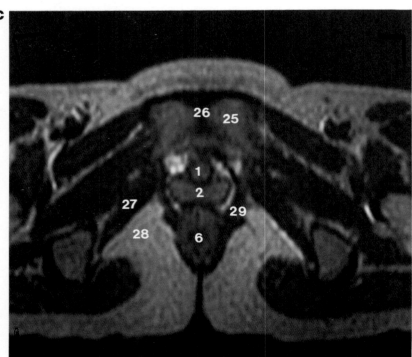

A–C Female pelvis. Axial MR images (T$_2$-weighted)

1	Urethra	22	Ovarian artery
2	Vagina	23	Broad ligament
3	Anterior	24	Round ligament
4	Posterior } fornix of vagina	25	Body of pubis
5	Lateral	26	Pubic symphysis
6	Rectum	27	Obturator internus muscle
7	Wall	28	Ischio-anal fossa
8	Endocervical canal } of cervix	29	Levator ani muscle
9	External os	30	Coccyx
10	Internal os	31	Sacrospinous ligament
11	Myometrium	32	Uterosacral ligament
12	Cavity } of uterus	33	Rectus abdominis muscle
13	Body	34	External iliac artery and vein
14	Fundus	35	Internal iliac artery and vein
15	Sigmoid colon	36	Sacrum
16	Bladder	37	Thecal sac
17	Ovary	38	Vestibule of vagina
18	Recto-uterine pouch	39	Labium majus
19	Anal canal	40	Clitoris
20	Ileum	41	Vesico-uterine pouch
21	Uterine artery		

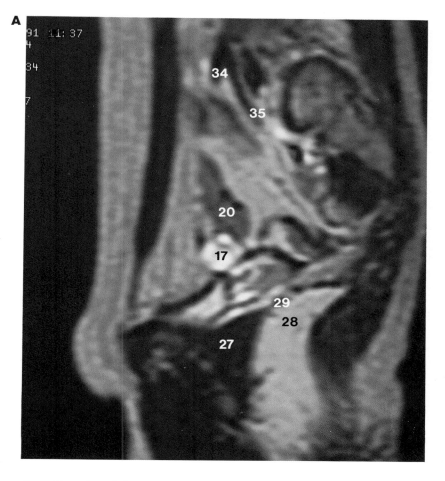

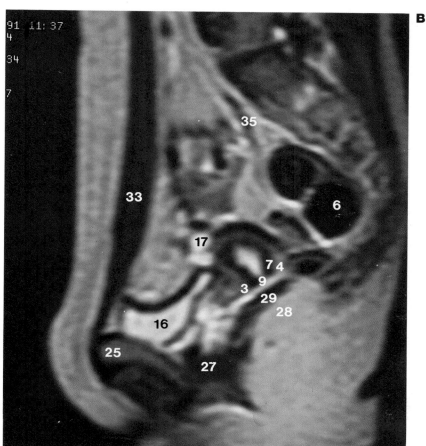

A–C Female pelvis. Sagittal MR images (T$_2$-weighted)

1	Urethra	22	Ovarian artery
2	Vagina	23	Broad ligament
3	Anterior	} fornix of vagina	24	Round ligament
4	Posterior		25	Body of pubis
5	Lateral		26	Pubic symphysis
6	Rectum		27	Obturator internus muscle
7	Wall	} of cervix	28	Ischio-anal fossa
8	Endocervical canal		29	Levator ani muscle
9	External os		30	Coccyx
10	Internal os		31	Sacrospinous ligament
11	Myometrium	} of uterus	32	Uterosacral ligament
12	Cavity		33	Rectus abdominis muscle
13	Body		34	External iliac artery and vein
14	Fundus		35	Internal iliac artery and vein
15	Sigmoid colon		36	Sacrum
16	Bladder		37	Thecal sac
17	Ovary		38	Vestibule of vagina
18	Recto-uterine pouch		39	Labium majus
19	Anal canal		40	Clitoris
20	Ileum		41	Vesico-uterine pouch
21	Uterine artery			

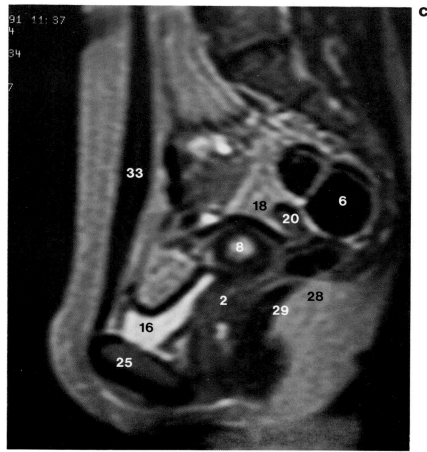

153

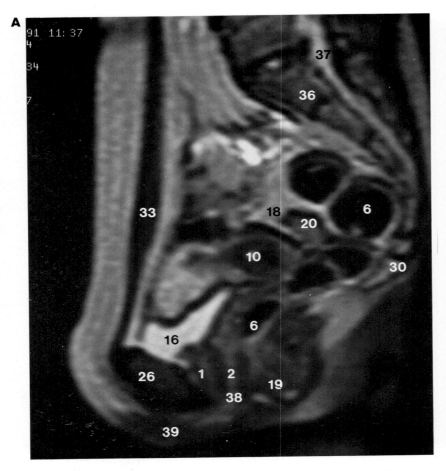

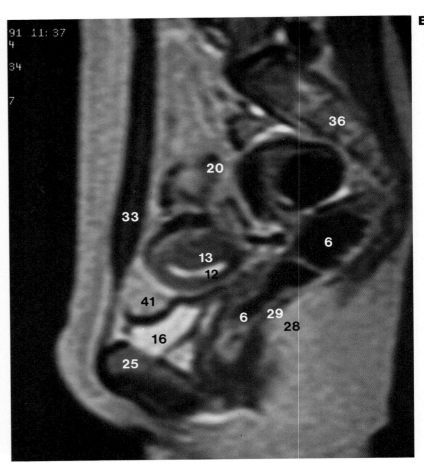

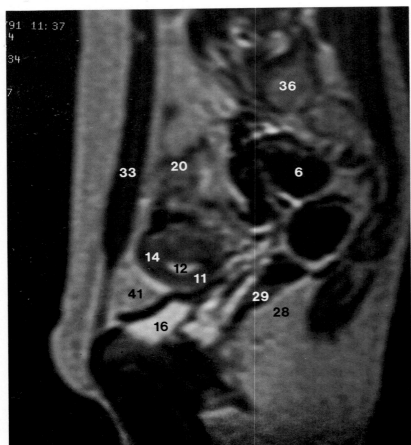

A–C Female pelvis. Sagittal MR images (T$_2$-weighted)

1	Urethra	22	Ovarian artery
2	Vagina	23	Broad ligament
3	Anterior ⎫	24	Round ligament
4	Posterior ⎬ fornix of vagina	25	Body of pubis
5	Lateral ⎭	26	Pubic symphysis
6	Rectum	27	Obturator internus muscle
7	Wall ⎫	28	Ischio-anal fossa
8	Endocervical canal ⎬ of cervix	29	Levator ani muscle
9	External os ⎪	30	Coccyx
10	Internal os ⎭	31	Sacrospinous ligament
11	Myometrium ⎫	32	Uterosacral ligament
12	Cavity ⎬ of uterus	33	Rectus abdominis muscle
13	Body ⎪	34	External iliac artery and vein
14	Fundus ⎭	35	Internal iliac artery and vein
15	Sigmoid colon	36	Sacrum
16	Bladder	37	Thecal sac
17	Ovary	38	Vestibule of vagina
18	Recto-uterine pouch	39	Labium majus
19	Anal canal	40	Clitoris
20	Ileum	41	Vesico-uterine pouch
21	Uterine artery		

A

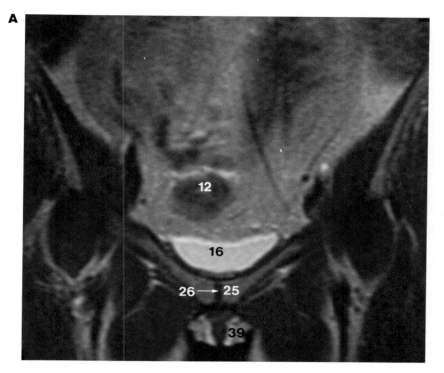

B

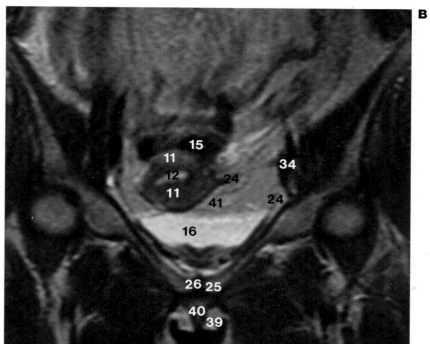

A–C Female pelvis. Coronal MR images (T$_2$-weighted)

C

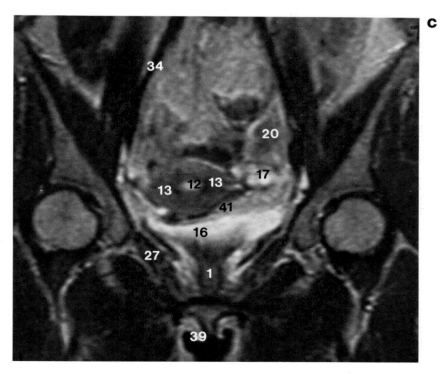

1	Urethra	22	Ovarian artery
2	Vagina	23	Broad ligament
3	Anterior	24	Round ligament
4	Posterior } fornix of vagina	25	Body of pubis
5	Lateral	26	Pubic symphysis
6	Rectum	27	Obturator internus muscle
7	Wall	28	Ischio-anal fossa
8	Endocervical canal } of cervix	29	Levator ani muscle
9	External os	30	Coccyx
10	Internal os	31	Sacrospinous ligament
11	Myometrium	32	Uterosacral ligament
12	Cavity } of uterus	33	Rectus abdominis muscle
13	Body	34	External iliac artery and vein
14	Fundus	35	Internal iliac artery and vein
15	Sigmoid colon	36	Sacrum
16	Bladder	37	Thecal sac
17	Ovary	38	Vestibule of vagina
18	Recto-uterine pouch	39	Labium majus
19	Anal canal	40	Clitoris
20	Ileum	41	Vesico-uterine pouch
21	Uterine artery		

A

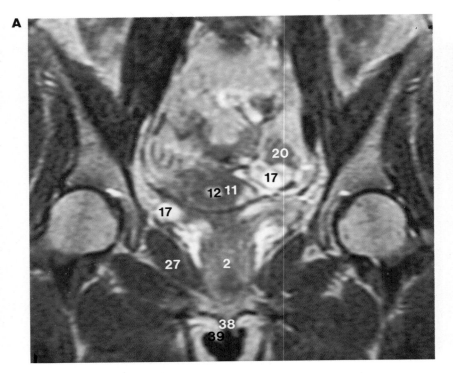

B

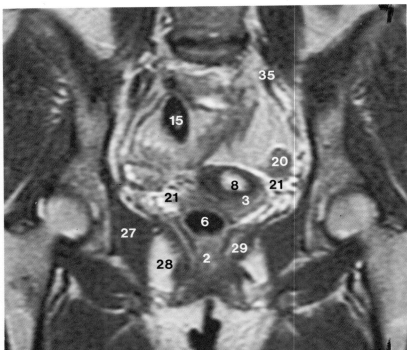

C

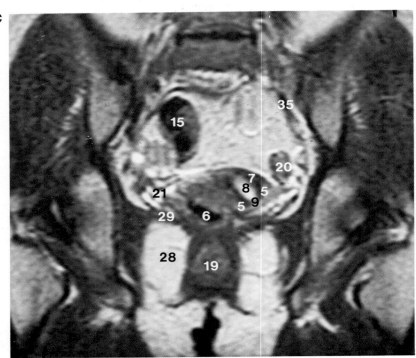

A—C Female pelvis. Coronal MR images (T$_2$-weighted)

1	Urethra	22	Ovarian artery
2	Vagina	23	Broad ligament
3	Anterior ⎫	24	Round ligament
4	Posterior ⎬ fornix of vagina	25	Body of pubis
5	Lateral ⎭	26	Pubic symphysis
6	Rectum	27	Obturator internus muscle
7	Wall ⎫	28	Ischio-anal fossa
8	Endocervical canal ⎬ of cervix	29	Levator ani muscle
9	External os ⎪	30	Coccyx
10	Internal os ⎭	31	Sacrospinous ligament
11	Myometrium ⎫	32	Uterosacral ligament
12	Cavity ⎬ of uterus	33	Rectus abdominis muscle
13	Body ⎪	34	External iliac artery and vein
14	Fundus ⎭	35	Internal iliac artery and vein
15	Sigmoid colon	36	Sacrum
16	Bladder	37	Thecal sac
17	Ovary	38	Vestibule of vagina
18	Recto-uterine pouch	39	Labium majus
19	Anal canal	40	Clitoris
20	Ileum	41	Vesico-uterine pouch
21	Uterine artery		

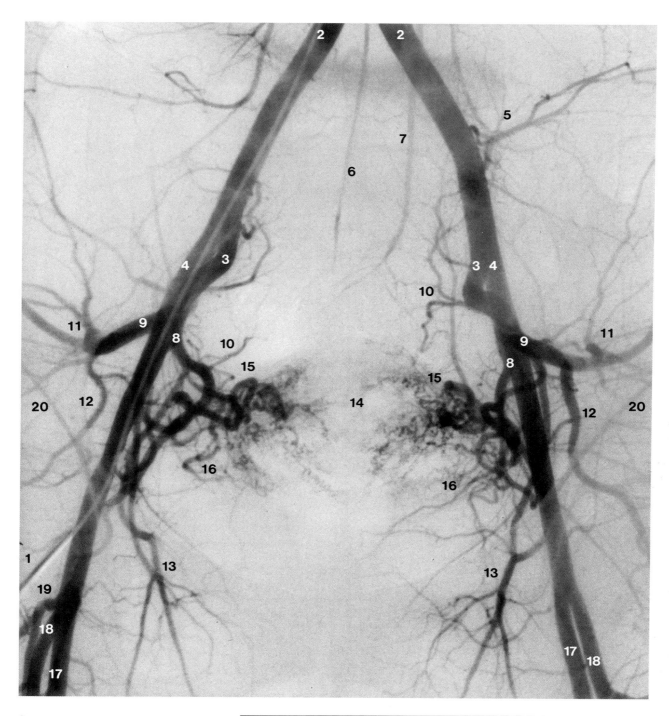

Subtracted pelvic arteriogram

This anteroposterior film of the pelvis demonstrates both the internal and the external iliac arteries and their branches. Many of the vessels are superimposed: to see them more clearly oblique projections could be obtained. The contrast medium injected into the arteries is excreted by the kidneys, and a full bladder may obscure the branches.

Selective catheterisation of the internal and external iliac arteries using a preshaped catheter gives better detail without superimposition of the vessels.

1	Catheter introduced into distal abdominal aorta via right femoral artery	10	Lateral sacral artery
2	Common iliac artery	11	Superior gluteal artery
3	Internal iliac artery	12	Inferior gluteal artery
4	External iliac artery	13	Obturator artery
5	Iliolumbar artery	14	Position of uterus
6	Median sacral artery	15	Uterine artery
7	Inferior mesenteric artery	16	Superior vesical artery
8	Anterior ⎫ trunk of internal iliac	17	Superficial femoral artery
9	Posterior ⎭ artery	18	Profunda femoris artery
		19	Lateral circumflex femoral artery
		20	Deep circumflex iliac artery

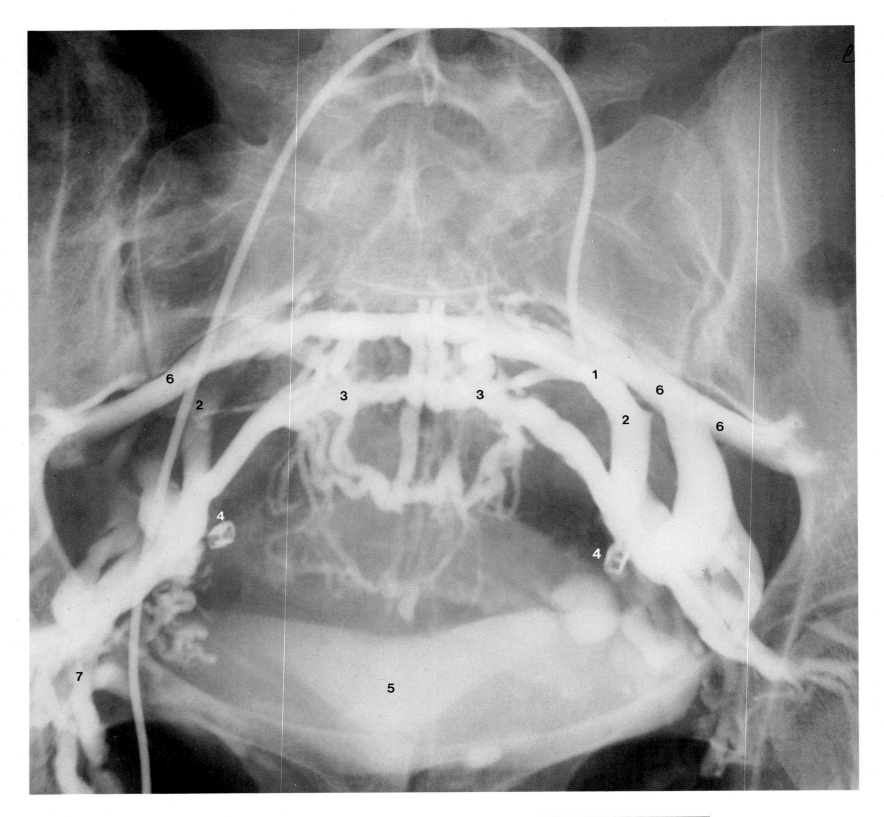

Female pelvic venogram

1   Catheter introduced via right femoral vein, with tip in left internal iliac vein
2   Anterior division of internal iliac vein
3   Sacral plexus of veins
4   Sterilisation clips
5   Bladder containing contrast medium
6   Gluteal veins
7   Obturator veins

A

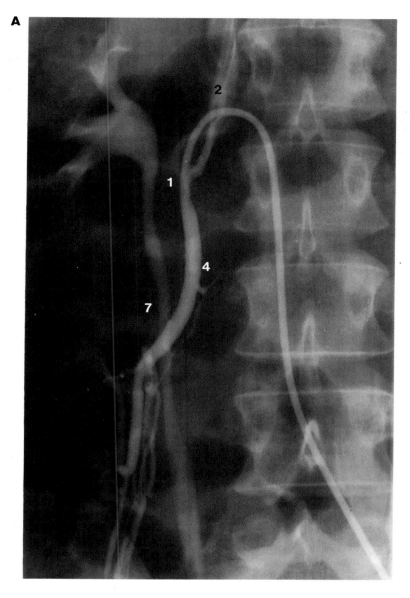

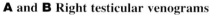

B

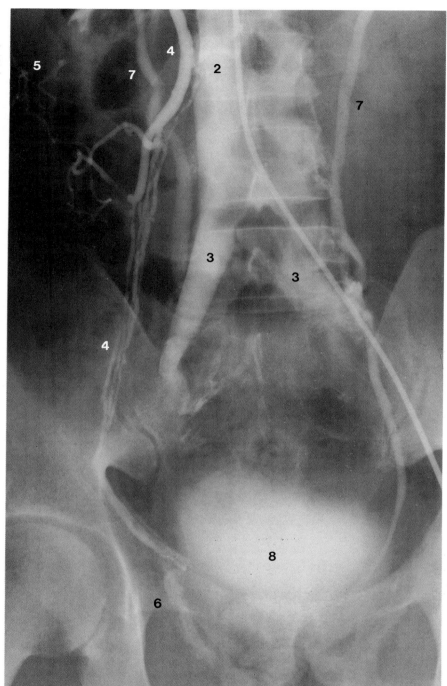

A and B Right testicular venograms

The gonadal veins drain into one or two main veins via a venous plexus. On the left, the main vein drains into the left renal vein. It may occasionally communicate with the inferior mesenteric vein and drain into the portal venous system. On the right, the main vein usually drains into the inferior vena cava directly (as in the cases illustrated), but it can drain into the right renal vein.

1	Tip of catheter in right testicular vein, introduced via left femoral vein
2	Inferior vena cava
3	Common iliac veins
4	Right testicular vein
5	Renal capsular veins
6	Pampiniform plexus of veins (undescended testis in inguinal canal)
7	Ureter
8	Bladder

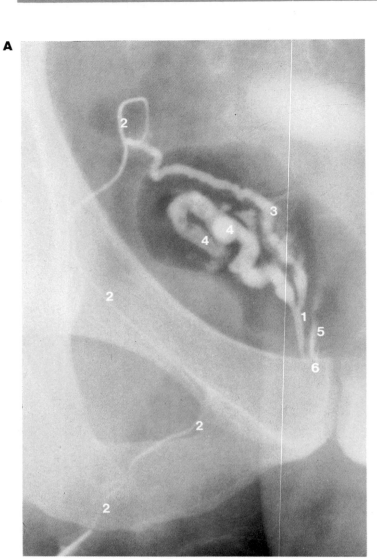

A Seminal vesiculogram

A Seminal vesiculogram

1	Right ejaculatory duct
2	Ductus deferens (vas deferens)
3	Ampulla of ductus deferens
4	Seminal vesicle
5	Left ejaculatory duct
6	Position of seminal colliculus (verumontanum)

B Male pelvis. Transverse transabdominal ultrasound image

1	Full urinary bladder
2	Seminal vesicle
3	Colonic gas

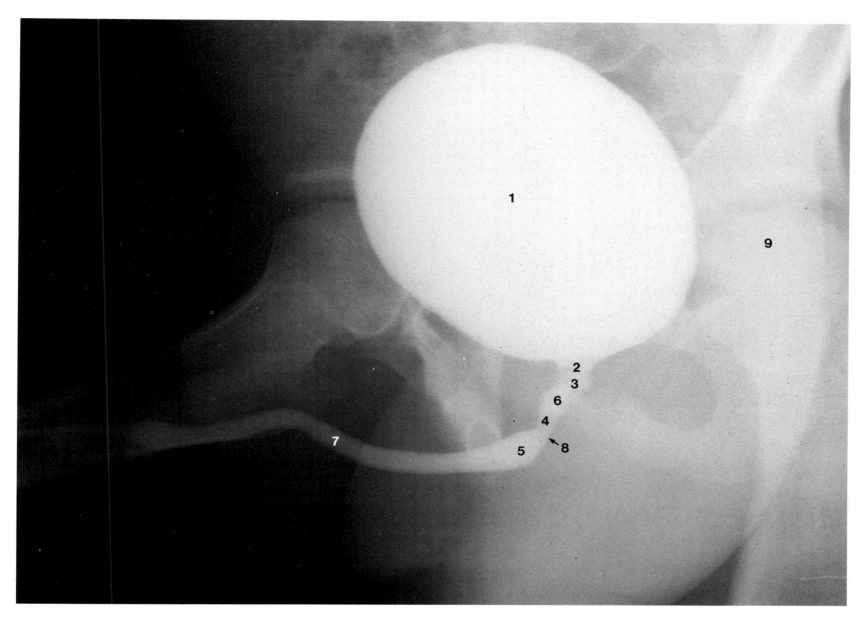

Male urethrogram. Oblique image

1 Contrast in urinary bladder	6 Seminal colliculus (verumontanum)
2 Neck of urinary bladder	7 Penile urethra
3 Prostatic urethra	8 External sphincter (sphincter urethrae)
4 Membranous urethra	9 Head of femur
5 Bulbous urethra	

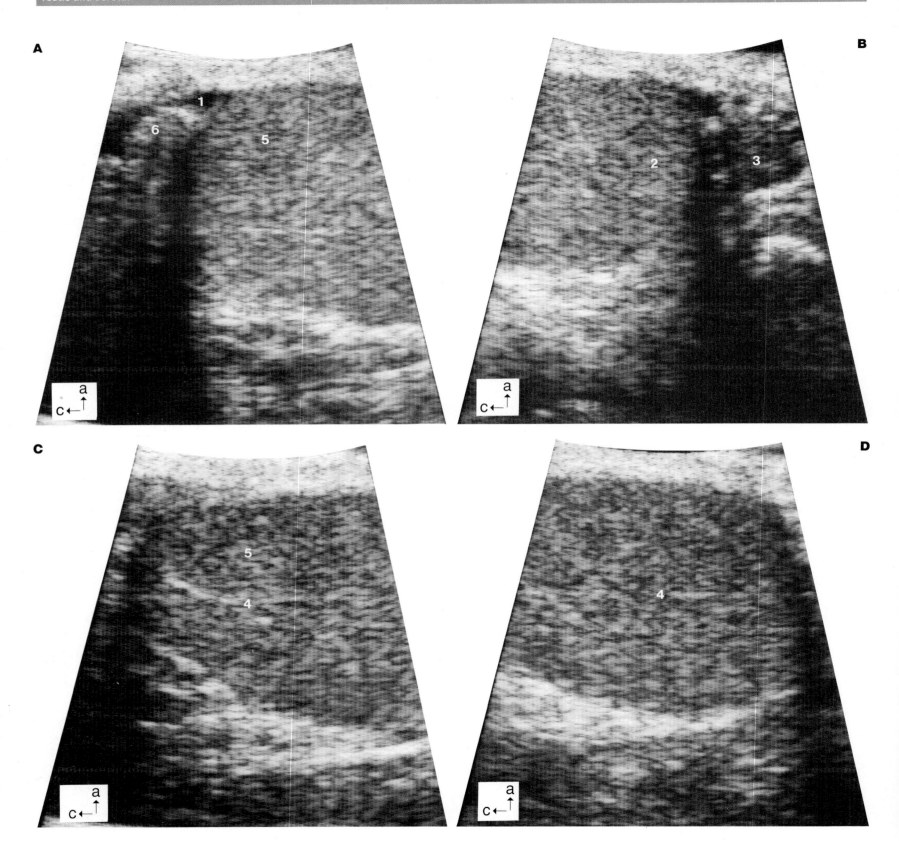

A–D Scrotum. Parasagittal ultrasound images (a = anterior, c = cranial)

1	Scrotal free fluid	4	Mediastinum testis
2	Lower pole of left testis	5	Upper pole of left testis
3	Tail of left epididymis	6	Head of left epididymis

Hysterosalpingograms,
A immediately after injection,
B some minutes after injection

1	Ampulla	} of uterine tube
2	Isthmus	
3	Cornu	
4	Fundus	} of uterus
5	Body	
6	Cervix	
7	Leech–Wilkinson cannula in cervix	
8	Contrast spillage into peritoneal cavity	

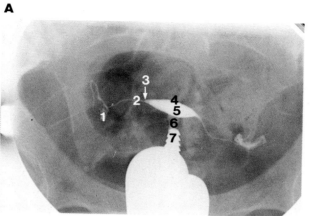

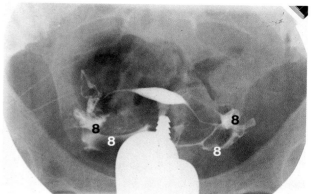

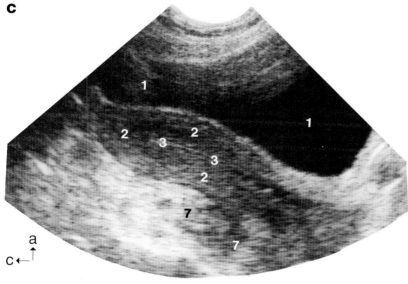

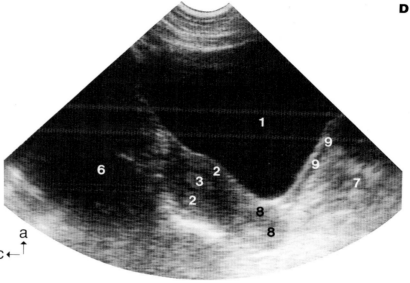

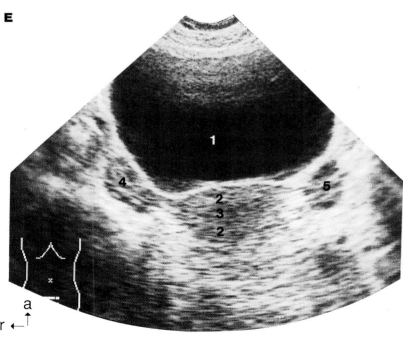

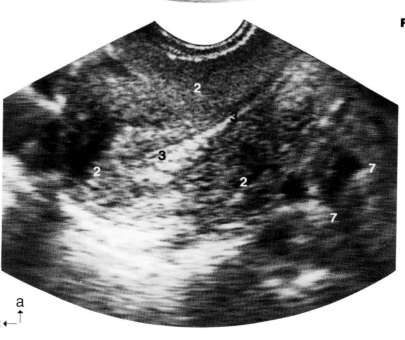

Female pelvis, C and **D** sagittal transabdominal ultrasound image, **E** transverse ultrasound image, **F** transvaginal ultrasound image (a = anterior, c = cranial, r = right)

1	Full urinary bladder	6	Sigmoid colonic shadowing
2	Myometrium	7	Rectal gas
3	Endometrium	8	Cervix of uterus
4	Right } ovary	9	Vagina
5	Left		

Lower limb

A Hip (for neck of femur).
Lateral projection

1	Acetabulum
2	Anterior inferior iliac spine
3	Ischial spine
4	Ischial tuberosity
5	Head of femur
6	Epiphysial line
7	Neck of femur
8	Greater ⎱ trochanter
9	Lesser ⎰
10	Intertrochanteric line

A

B Hip. Lateral projection

1	Acetabulum
2	Head ⎫
3	Greater trochanter ⎬ of femur
4	Intertrochanteric crest
5	Lesser trochanter ⎭
6	Ischial spine
7	Ischial tuberosity
8	Obturator foramen
9	Superior ramus of pubis
10	Pubic symphysis

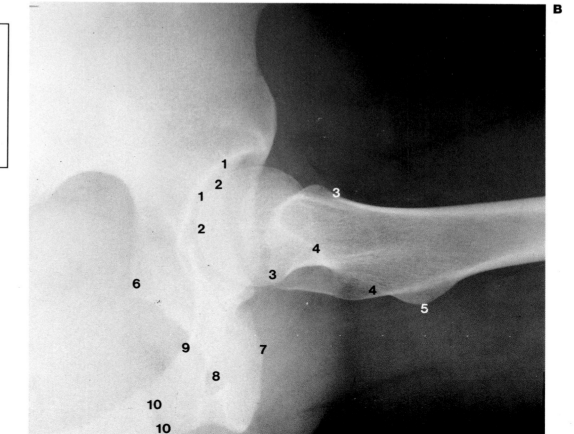

B

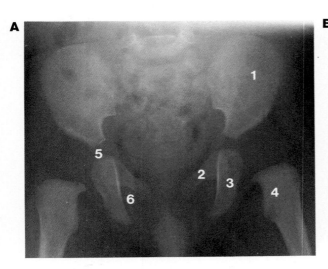

A

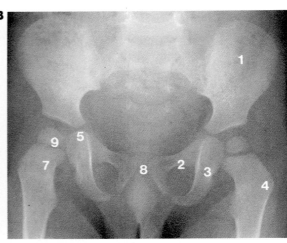

B

Pelvis, **A** of a 2-month-old boy, **B** of a 1-year-old boy, **C** of an 11-year-old boy. Anteroposterior projections

1	Ilium
2	Pubis
3	Ischium
4	Femur
5	Triradiate cartilage
6	Unossified junction between ischium and pubis
7	Neck of femur
8	Pubic symphysis
9	Centre for head of femur (femoral capital epiphysis)
10	Centre for greater } trochanter
11	Centre for lesser

C

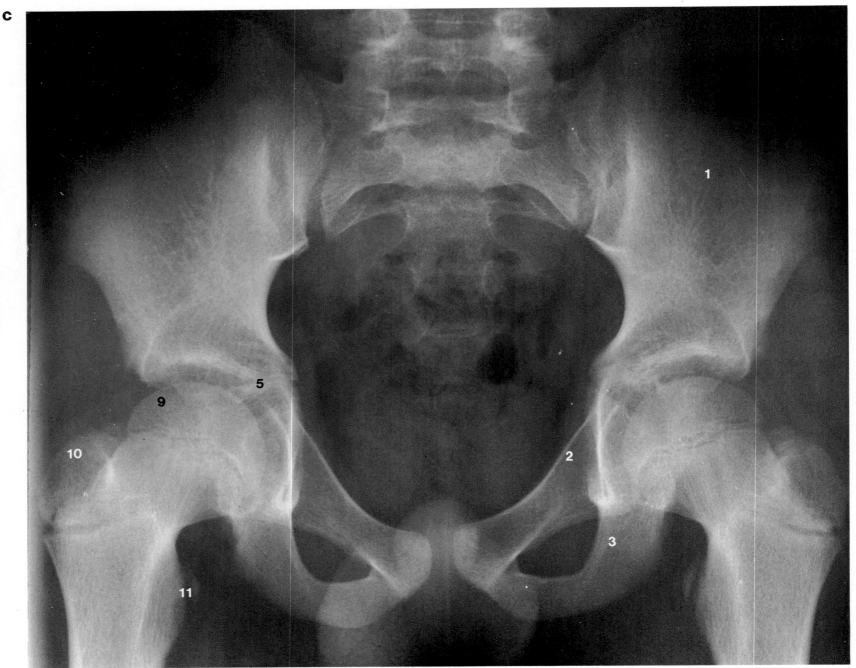

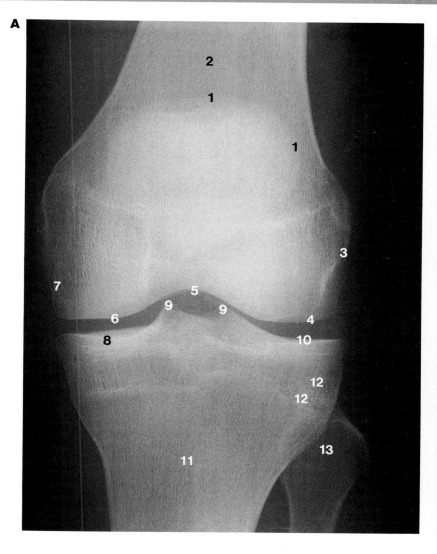

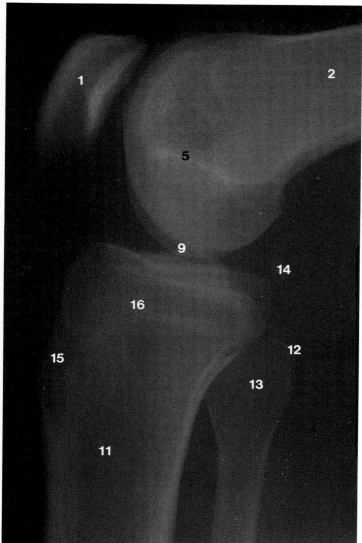

Knee, A anteroposterior projection, **B** lateral projection

C Patella. Inferosuperior (skyline) projection

1	Patella
2	Femur
3	Lateral epicondyle ⎫ of femur
4	Lateral condyle ⎭
5	Intercondylar fossa
6	Medial condyle ⎫ of femur
7	Medial epicondyle ⎭
8	Medial condyle of tibia
9	Tubercles of intercondylar eminence
10	Lateral condyle of tibia
11	Tibia
12	Apex (styloid process) ⎫ of fibula
13	Head ⎭
14	Fabella
15	Tuberosity of tibia
16	Epiphysial line

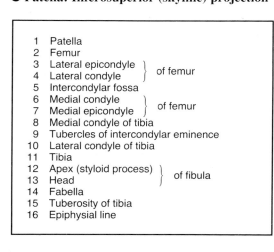

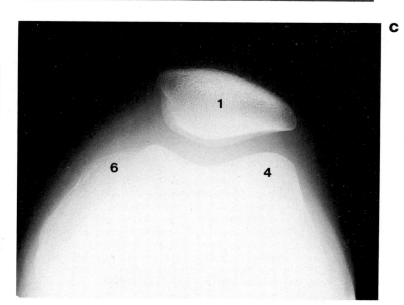

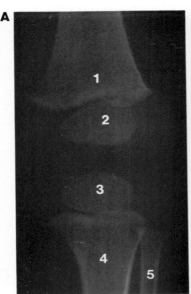

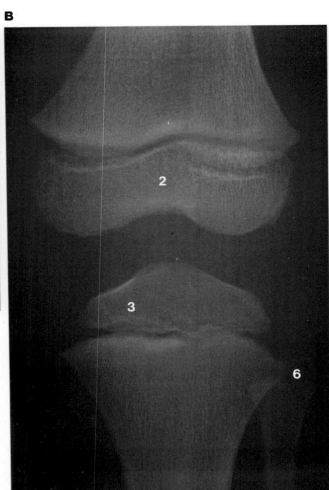

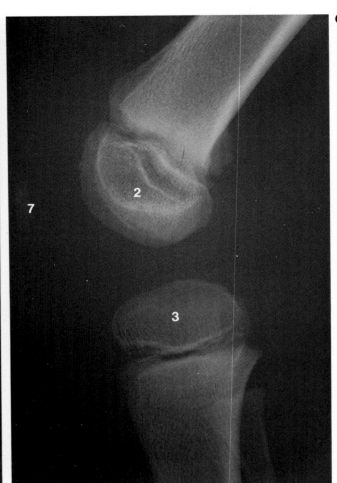

Knee, **A** of a 1-year-old boy,
B and **C** of a 6-year-old boy,
D and **E** of a 12-year-old boy

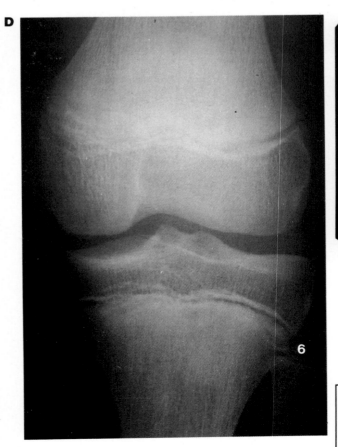

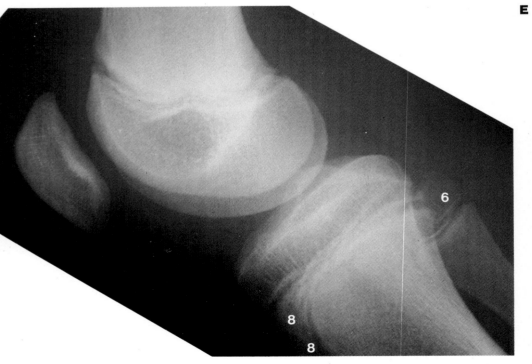

1	Femur	5	Fibula
2	Centre for distal femur	6	Centre for head of fibula
3	Centre for proximal tibia	7	Centre for patella
4	Tibia	8	Antero-inferior extension of proximal tibial centre for tuberosity of tibia

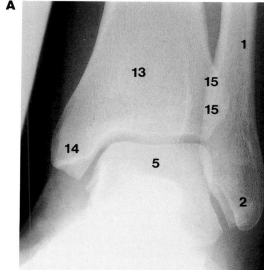

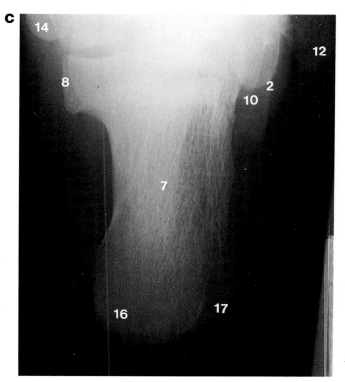

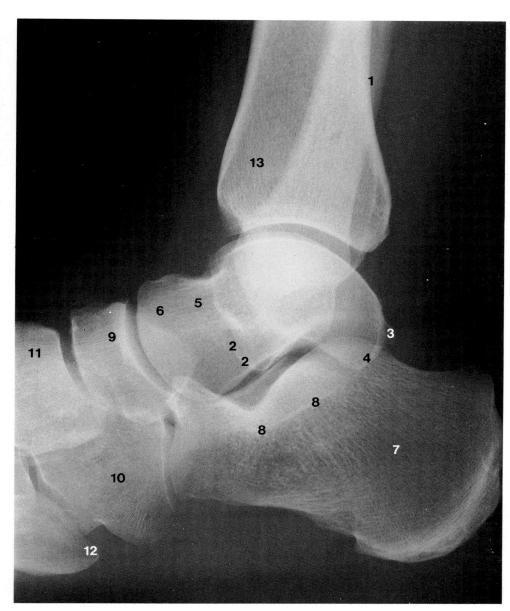

Ankle, **A** anteroposterior projection,
B lateral projection

C Calcaneus. Axial projection

1	Fibula	10	Cuboid
2	Lateral malleolus of fibula	11	Lateral cuneiform
3	Lateral } tubercle of talus	12	Tuberosity of base of fifth metatarsal
4	Medial	13	Tibia
5	Talus	14	Medial malleolus of tibia
6	Head of talus	15	Region of inferior tibiofibular joint
7	Calcaneus	16	Medial } process of calcaneus
8	Sustentaculum tali of calcaneus	17	Lateral
9	Navicular		

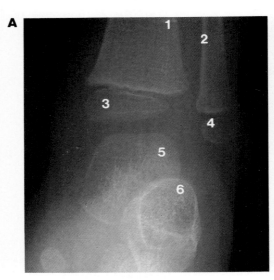

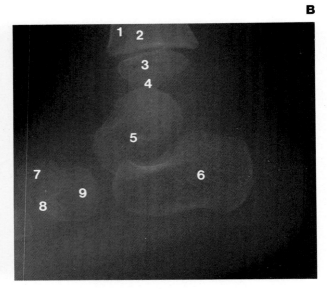

Ankle, **A** and **B** of a 3-year-old boy, **C** and **D** of a 5-year-old boy, **E** and **F** of a 13-year-old boy

1	Tibia
2	Fibula
3	Centre for distal tibia
4	Centre for distal fibula
5	Talus
6	Calcaneus
7	Lateral ⎫
8	Intermediate ⎬ cuneiform
9	Cuboid
10	Navicular
11	Centre for posterior aspect of calcaneus

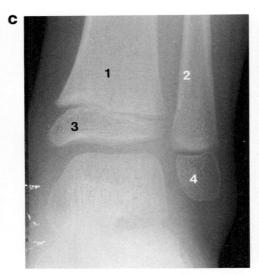

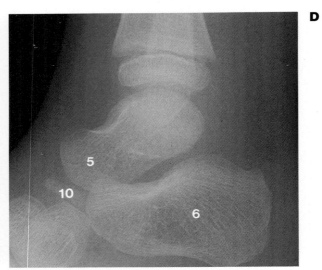

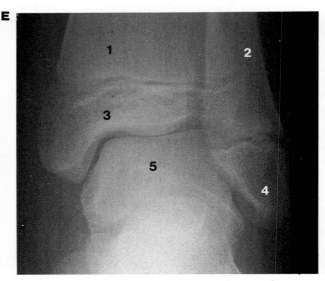

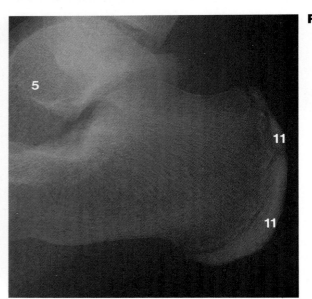

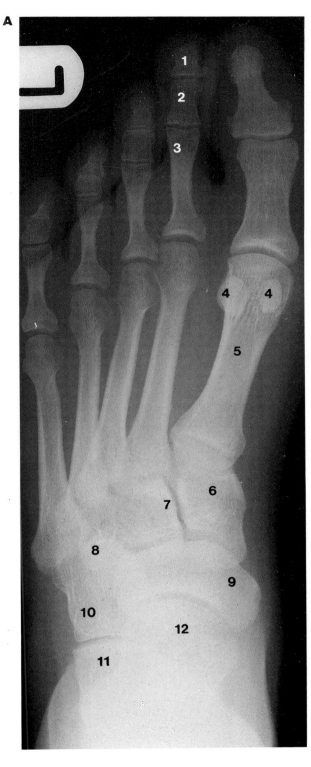

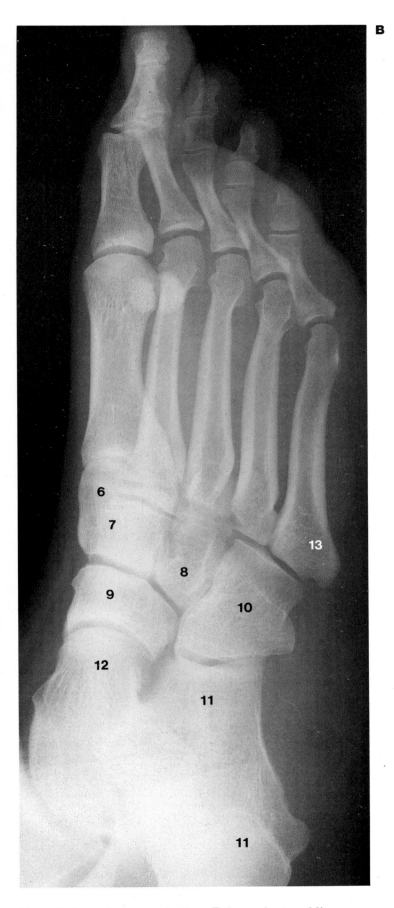

1 Distal ⎫
2 Middle ⎬ phalanx of second toe
3 Proximal ⎭
4 Sesamoid bones in flexor hallucis brevis muscle
5 First metatarsal
6 Medial   ⎫
7 Intermediate ⎬ cuneiform
8 Lateral   ⎭
9 Navicular
10 Cuboid
11 Calcaneus
12 Talus
13 Tuberosity of base of fifth metatarsal

Foot, A dorsoplantar projection, B dorsoplantar oblique projection

A

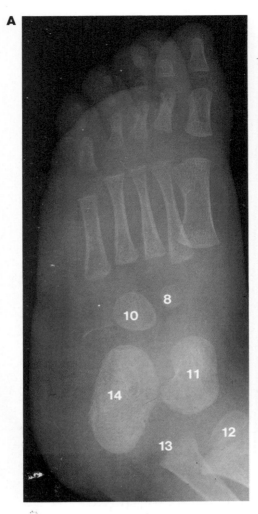

B

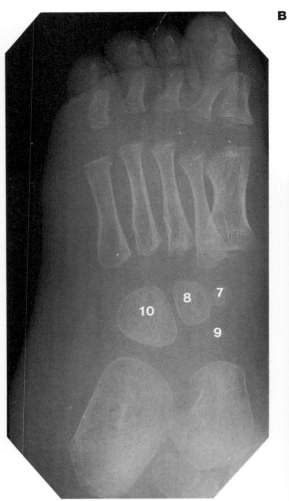

D

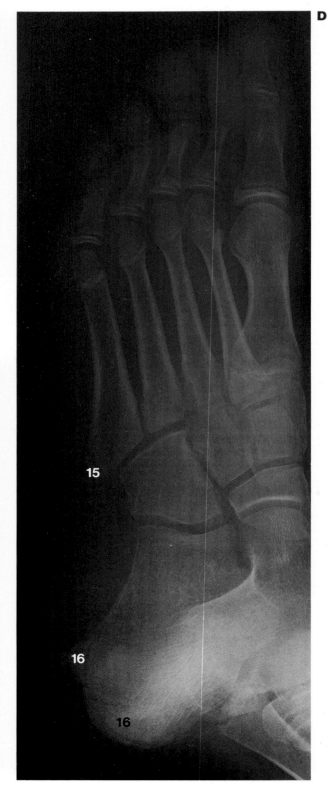

Foot, **A** of a 1-year-old boy, **B** of a
3-year-old boy, **C** of a 5-year-old boy,
D of a 14-year-old boy

C

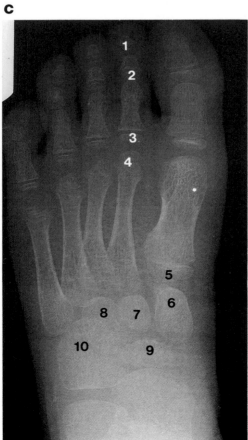

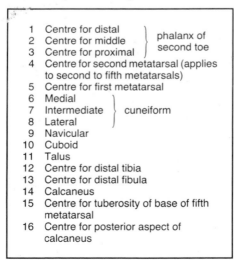

1	Centre for distal	⎫
2	Centre for middle	⎬ phalanx of
3	Centre for proximal	⎭ second toe
4	Centre for second metatarsal (applies to second to fifth metatarsals)	
5	Centre for first metatarsal	
6	Medial	⎫
7	Intermediate	⎬ cuneiform
8	Lateral	⎭
9	Navicular	
10	Cuboid	
11	Talus	
12	Centre for distal tibia	
13	Centre for distal fibula	
14	Calcaneus	
15	Centre for tuberosity of base of fifth metatarsal	
16	Centre for posterior aspect of calcaneus	

A

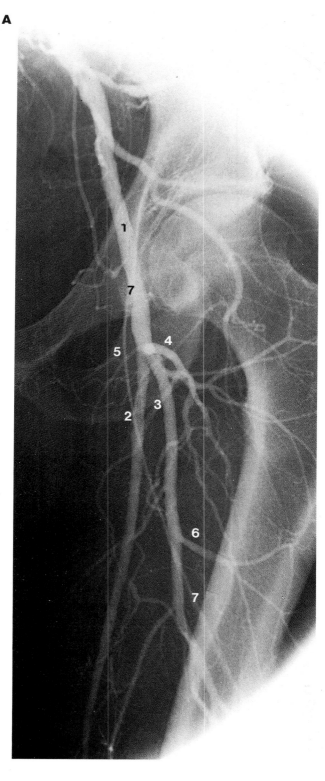

A Femoral arteriogram

The femoropopliteal and tibial arteries are imaged by catheterising the distal abdominal aorta and injecting contrast medium. The column of contrast is then followed as it passes down the legs. If only one leg is to be imaged, an injection into the ipsilateral femoral artery suffices. The external iliac artery continues as the common femoral artery, which originates deep to the inguinal ligament, dividing into the superficial and deep (profunda) femoral arteries. An oblique view is often useful to image the femoral bifurcation and to identify atheroma at the origins of these vessels.

1	Common femoral artery
2	Superficial femoral artery
3	Profunda femoris artery
4	Lateral circumflex femoral artery
5	Medial circumflex femoral artery
6	Perforating artery
7	Catheter introduced into distal abdominal aorta via left femoral artery

B Popliteal arteriogram

The superficial femoral artery becomes the popliteal artery as it passes through the hiatus in the adductor magnus muscle. The popliteal artery terminates at the lower border of the popliteus muscle, dividing into the anterior and posterior tibial arteries.

1	Popliteal artery
2	Superior lateral genicular artery
3	Superior medial genicular artery
4	Inferior medial genicular artery
5	Inferior lateral genicular artery
6	Anterior tibial artery
7	Posterior tibial artery
8	Peroneal artery
9	Muscular branches of posterior tibial artery
10	Muscular branches of anterior tibial artery

B

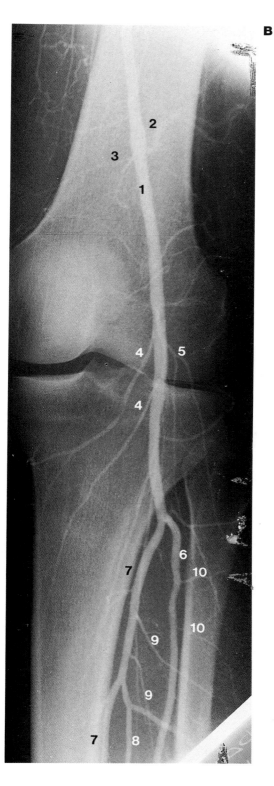

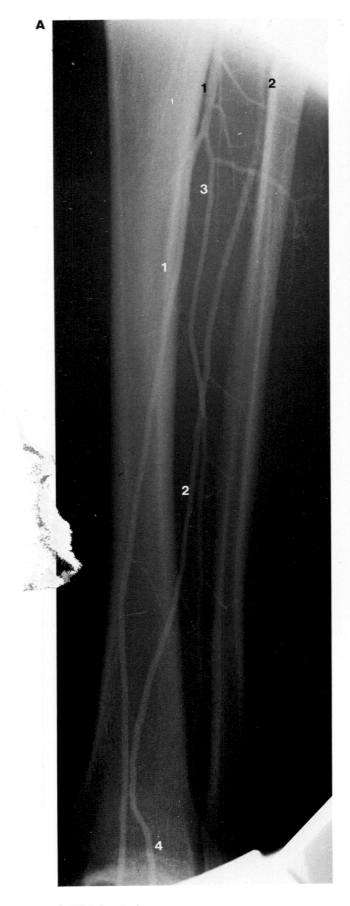

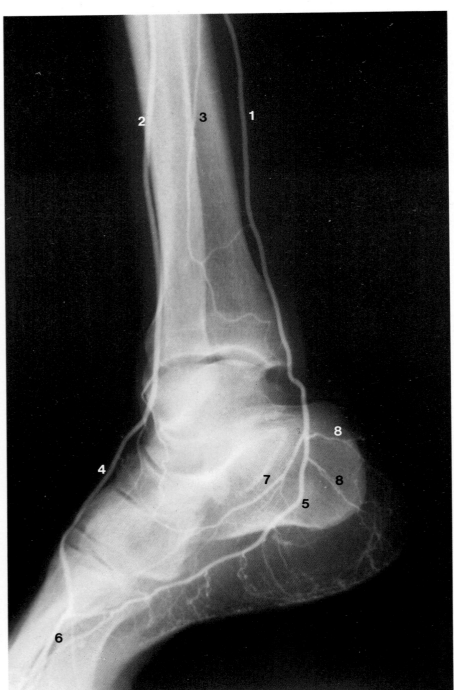

B Foot arteriogram. Lateral image

1	Posterior tibial artery
2	Anterior tibial artery
3	Peroneal artery
4	Dorsalis pedis artery
5	Lateral plantar artery
6	Plantar arch
7	Medial plantar artery
8	Medial calcaneal artery

A Tibial arteriogram

A

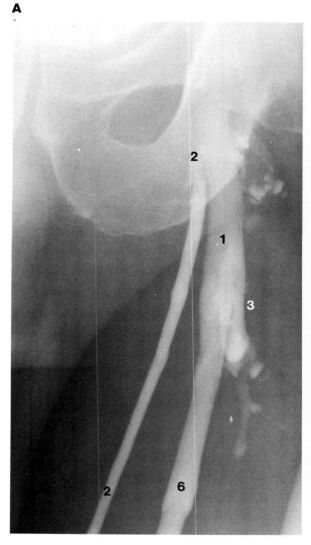

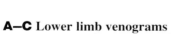

B

C

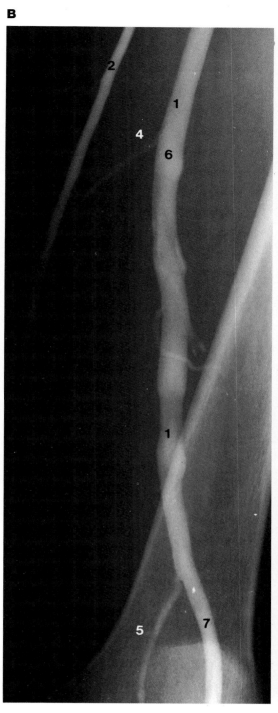

A–C Lower limb venograms

1	Femoral vein
2	Great (long) saphenous vein
3	Lateral circumflex vein
4	Perforating vein
5	Muscular tributary of femoral vein
6	Venous valves
7	Popliteal vein
8	Anterior tibial vein
9	Posterior tibial veins

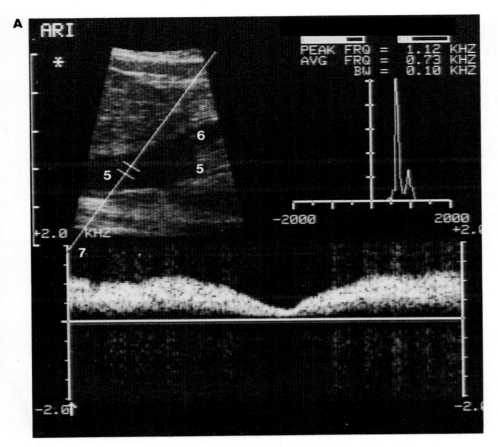

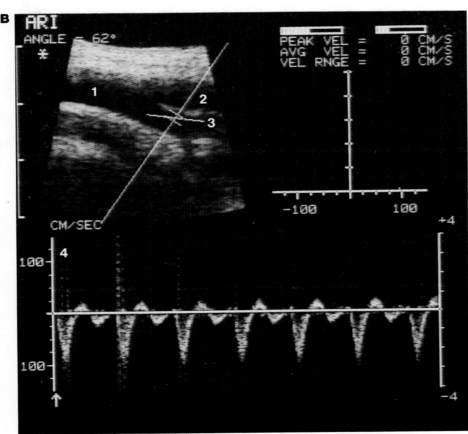

Lower limb vasculature, **A** and **B** oblique ultrasound images immediately inferior to the left inguinal ligament, **C** sagittal ultrasound image of the popliteal fossa

1	Femoral artery
2	Superficial femoral artery
3	Profunda femoris artery
4	Velocity wave form (profunda femoris artery, pulsed – Doppler study)
5	Femoral vein
6	Great (long) saphenous vein
7	Velocity wave form (femoral vein, pulsed – Doppler study)
8	Distal femur
9	Proximal tibia
10	Tibiofemoral joint
11	Popliteal artery
12	Popliteal vein

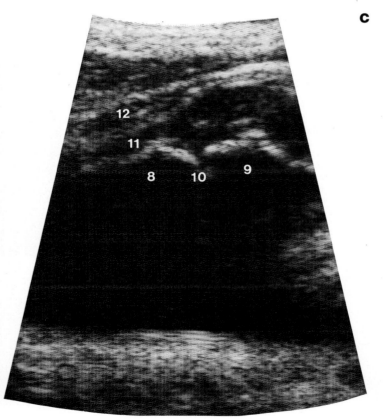

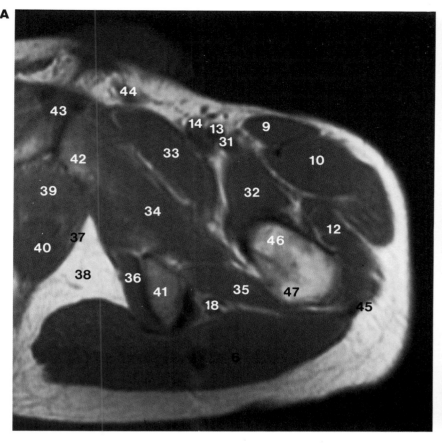

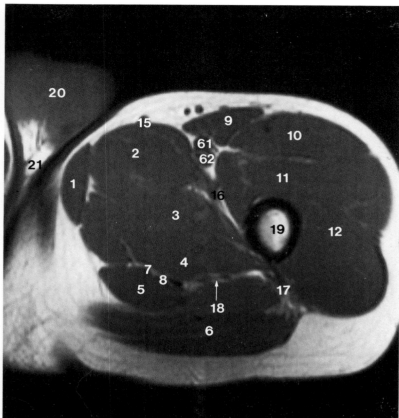

A—C Thigh. Axial MR images (T₁-weighted)

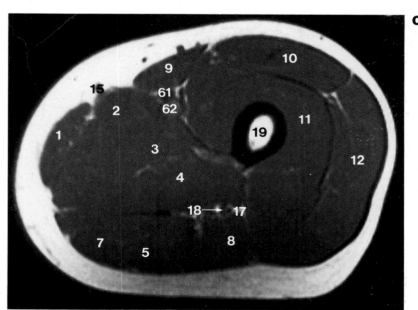

1 Gracilis muscle	33 Pectineus muscle
2 Adductor longus muscle	34 Obturator externus muscle
3 Adductor brevis muscle	35 Quadratus femoris muscle
4 Adductor magnus muscle	36 Obturator internus muscle
5 Semitendinosus muscle	37 Levator ani muscle
6 Gluteus maximus muscle	38 Ischio-anal fossa
7 Semimembranosus muscle	39 Prostate
8 Biceps femoris muscle	40 Anal canal
9 Sartorius muscle	41 Ischial tuberosity
10 Rectus femoris muscle	42 Inferior ramus of pubis
11 Vastus intermedius muscle	43 Pubic symphysis
12 Vastus lateralis muscle	44 Spermatic cord
13 Femoral artery	45 Iliotibial tract
14 Femoral vein	46 Neck of femur
15 Great (long) saphenous vein	47 Intertrochanteric ridge
16 Profunda femoris artery	48 Superior ramus of pubis
17 Lateral intermuscular septum	49 Bladder
18 Sciatic nerve	50 Corpus cavernosum
19 Femur	51 Corpus spongiosum
20 Testis	52 Greater ⎫ trochanter of femur
21 Scrotum	53 Lesser ⎭
22 Vastus medialis muscle	54 Gluteus medius muscle
23 Long ⎫ head of biceps	55 Head of femur
24 Short ⎭ femoris muscle	56 Acetabulum
25 Tendon of rectus femoris muscle	57 Rectum
26 Tendon of quadriceps muscle	58 Ischium
27 Tendon of semitendinosus	59 Piriformis muscle
muscle	60 Gemellus muscle
28 Popliteal artery	61 Superficial femoral artery
29 Popliteal vein	62 Superficial femoral vein
30 Tendon of gracilis muscle	63 Medial ⎫ head of
31 Femoral nerve	64 Lateral ⎭ gastrocnemius muscle
32 Iliopsoas muscle	65 Patella

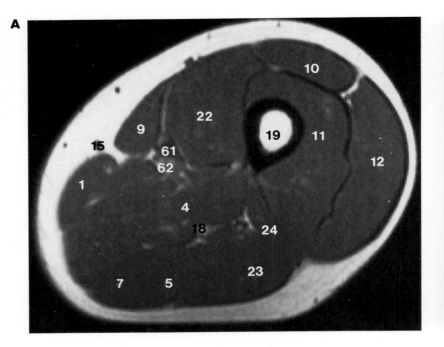

A **B**

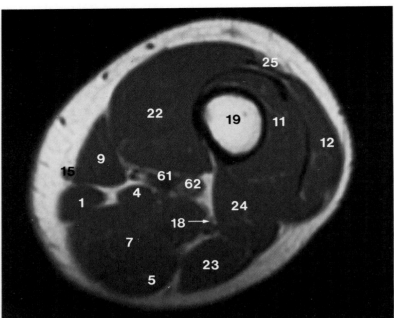

A—C Thigh. Axial MR images (T₁-weighted)

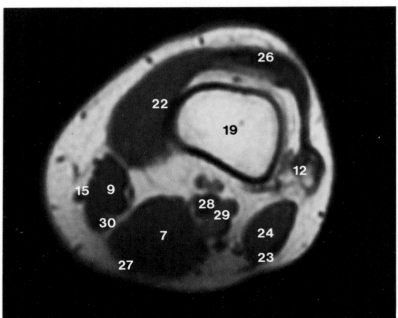

C

D—I Thigh. Sagittal MR images (T₁-weighted)

1	Gracilis muscle	32	Iliopsoas muscle
2	Adductor longus muscle	33	Pectineus muscle
3	Adductor brevis muscle	34	Obturator externus muscle
4	Adductor magnus muscle	35	Quadratus femoris muscle
5	Semitendinosus muscle	36	Obturator internus muscle
6	Gluteus maximus muscle	37	Levator ani muscle
7	Semimembranosus muscle	38	Ischio-anal fossa
8	Biceps femoris muscle	39	Prostate
9	Sartorius muscle	40	Anal canal
10	Rectus femoris muscle	41	Ischial tuberosity
11	Vastus intermedius muscle	42	Inferior ramus of pubis
12	Vastus lateralis muscle	43	Pubic symphysis
13	Femoral artery	44	Spermatic cord
14	Femoral vein	45	Iliotibial tract
15	Great (long) saphenous vein	46	Neck of femur
16	Profunda femoris artery	47	Intertrochanteric ridge
17	Lateral intermuscular septum	48	Superior ramus of pubis
18	Sciatic nerve	49	Bladder
19	Femur	50	Corpus cavernosum
20	Testis	51	Corpus spongiosum
21	Scrotum	52	Greater | trochanter
22	Vastus medialis muscle	53	Lesser | of femur
23	Long | head of biceps	54	Gluteus medius muscle
24	Short | femoris muscle	55	Head of femur
25	Tendon of rectus femoris muscle	56	Acetabulum
		57	Rectum
26	Tendon of quadriceps muscle	58	Ischium
		59	Piriformis muscle
27	Tendon of semitendinosus muscle	60	Gemellus muscle
		61	Superficial femoral artery
28	Popliteal artery	62	Superficial femoral vein
29	Popliteal vein	63	Medial | head of
30	Tendon of gracilis muscle	64	Lateral | gastrocnemius muscle
31	Femoral nerve	65	Patella

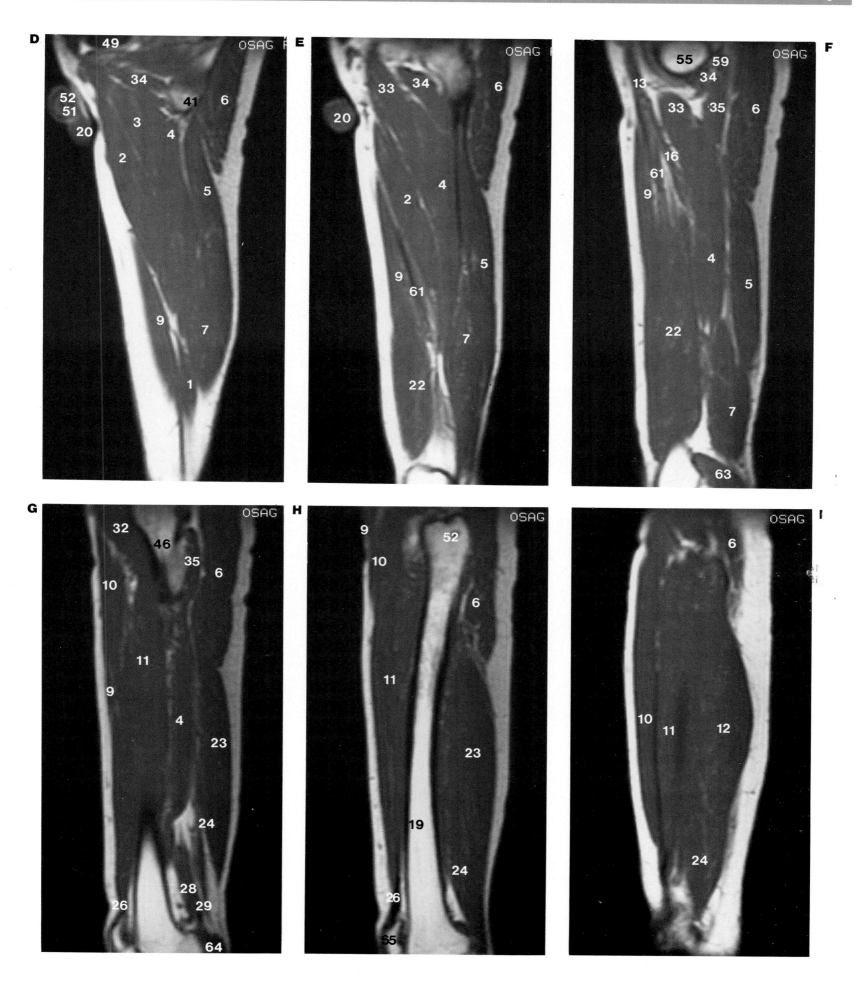

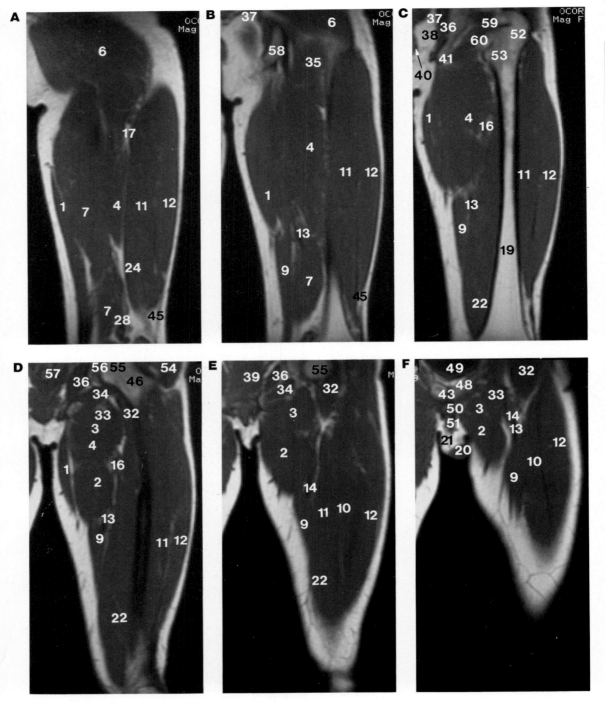

1 Gracilis muscle
2 Adductor longus muscle
3 Adductor brevis muscle
4 Adductor magnus muscle
5 Semitendinosus muscle
6 Gluteus maximus muscle
7 Semimembranosus muscle
8 Biceps femoris muscle
9 Sartorius muscle
10 Rectus femoris muscle
11 Vastus intermedius muscle
12 Vastus lateralis muscle
13 Femoral artery
14 Femoral vein
15 Great (long) saphenous vein
16 Profunda femoris artery
17 Lateral intermuscular septum
18 Sciatic nerve
19 Femur
20 Testis
21 Scrotum
22 Vastus medialis muscle
23 Long } head of biceps
24 Short } femoris muscle
25 Tendon of rectus femoris muscle
26 Tendon of quadriceps muscle
27 Tendon of semitendinosus muscle
28 Popliteal artery
29 Popliteal vein
30 Tendon of gracilis muscle
31 Femoral nerve
32 Iliopsoas muscle
33 Pectineus muscle
34 Obturator externus muscle
35 Quadratus femoris muscle
36 Obturator internus muscle
37 Levator ani muscle
38 Ischio-anal fossa
39 Prostate
40 Anal canal
41 Ischial tuberosity
42 Inferior ramus of pubis
43 Pubic symphysis
44 Spermatic cord
45 Iliotibial tract
46 Neck of femur
47 Intertrochanteric ridge
48 Superior ramus of pubis
49 Bladder
50 Corpus cavernosum
51 Corpus spongiosum
52 Greater }
53 Lesser } trochanter of femur
54 Gluteus medius muscle
55 Head of femur
56 Acetabulum
57 Rectum
58 Ischium
59 Piriformis muscle
60 Gemellus muscle
61 Superficial femoral artery
62 Superficial femoral vein
63 Medial }
64 Lateral } head of gastrocnemius muscle
65 Patella

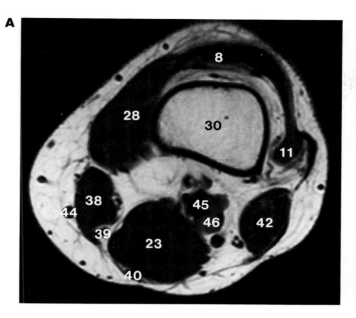

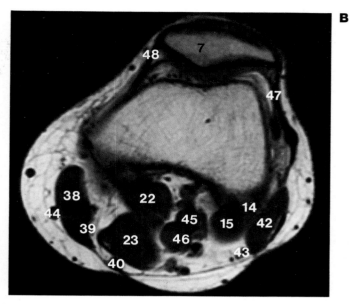

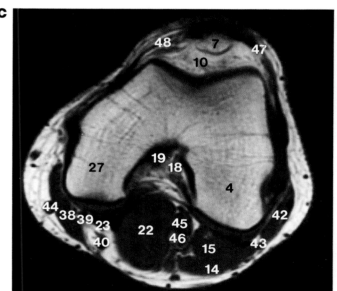

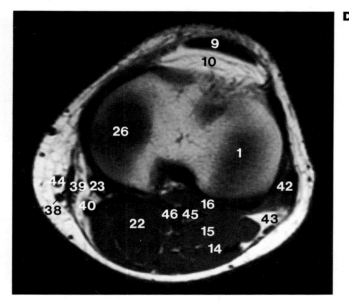

A—E Knee. Axial MR images (T$_1$-weighted)

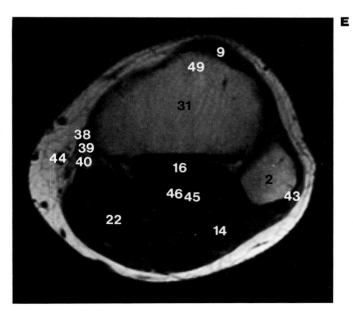

1	Lateral condyle of tibia	26	Medial condyle of tibia
2	Head of fibula	27	Medial condyle of femur
3	Tibiofibular joint	28	Vastus medialis muscle
4	Lateral condyle of femur	29	Posterior meniscofemoral ligament
5	Anterior ⎱ horn of lateral meniscus	30	Femur
6	Posterior ⎰	31	Tibia
7	Patella	32	Iliotibial tract
8	Tendon of quadriceps muscle	33	Tibialis anterior muscle
9	Patellar tendon	34	Medial collateral ligament
10	Infrapatellar fat pad	35	Medial ⎱ meniscus
11	Vastus lateralis muscle	36	Lateral ⎰
12	Short head of biceps femoris muscle	37	Lateral collateral ligament
13	Superior lateral genicular artery	38	Sartorius muscle
14	Lateral head of gastrocnemius muscle	39	Gracilis muscle
15	Plantaris muscle	40	Tendon of semitendinosus muscle
16	Popliteus muscle	41	Soleus muscle
17	Long head of biceps femoris muscle	42	Biceps femoris muscle
18	Anterior cruciate ligament	43	Common peroneal nerve
19	Posterior cruciate ligament	44	Great saphenous vein
20	Intercondylar notch	45	Popliteal artery
21	Popliteal artery and vein	46	Popliteal vein
22	Medial head of gastrocnemius muscle	47	Lateral ⎱ patellar retinaculum
23	Semimembranosus muscle	48	Medial ⎰
24	Anterior ⎱ horn of medial meniscus	49	Tibial tubercle
25	Posterior ⎰		

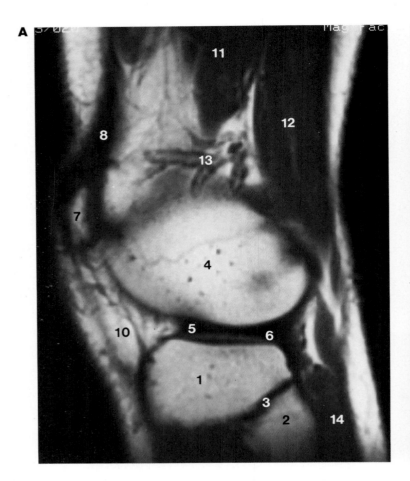

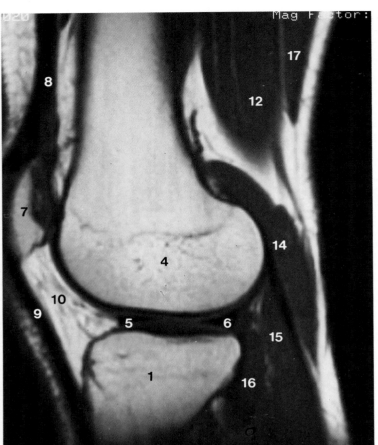

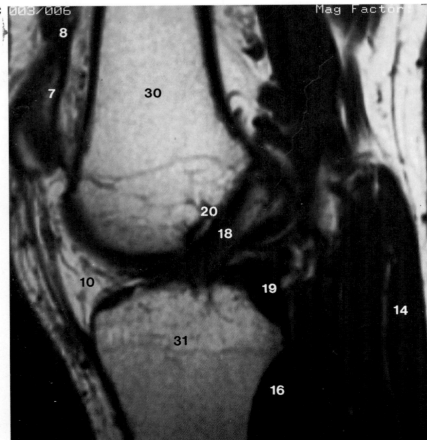

A—F Knee. Sagittal MR images (T₁-weighted)

1 Lateral condyle of tibia
2 Head of fibula
3 Tibiofibular joint
4 Lateral condyle of femur
5 Anterior ⎫
6 Posterior ⎬ horn of lateral meniscus
7 Patella
8 Tendon of quadriceps muscle
9 Patellar tendon
10 Infrapatellar fat pad
11 Vastus lateralis muscle
12 Short head of biceps femoris muscle
13 Superior lateral genicular artery
14 Lateral head of gastrocnemius muscle
15 Plantaris muscle
16 Popliteus muscle
17 Long head of biceps femoris muscle
18 Anterior cruciate ligament
19 Posterior cruciate ligament
20 Intercondylar notch
21 Popliteal artery and vein
22 Medial head of gastrocnemius muscle
23 Semimembranosus muscle
24 Anterior ⎫
25 Posterior ⎬ horn of medial meniscus

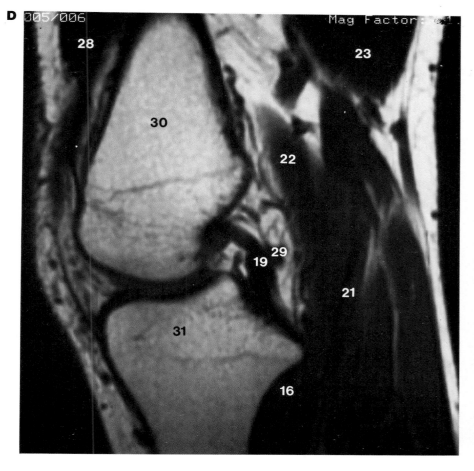

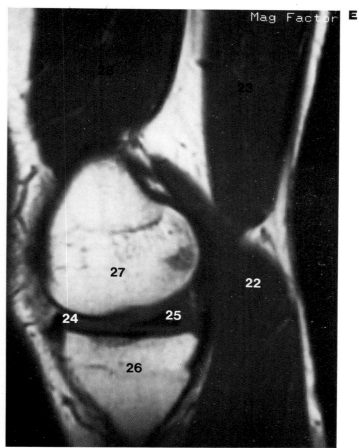

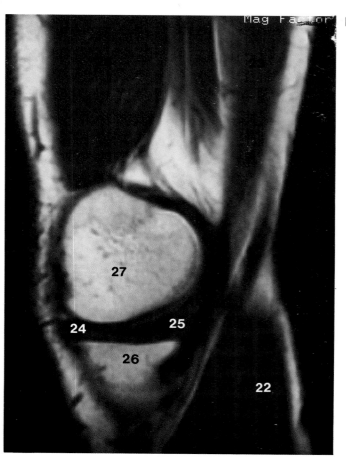

26	Medial condyle of tibia
27	Medial condyle of femur
28	Vastus medialis muscle
29	Posterior meniscofemoral ligament
30	Femur
31	Tibia
32	Iliotibial tract
33	Tibialis anterior muscle
34	Medial collateral ligament
35	Medial meniscus
36	Lateral
37	Lateral collateral ligament
38	Sartorius muscle
39	Gracilis muscle
40	Tendon of semitendinosus muscle
41	Soleus muscle
42	Biceps femoris muscle
43	Common peroneal nerve
44	Great saphenous vein
45	Popliteal artery
46	Popliteal vein
47	Lateral patellar retinaculum
48	Medial
49	Tibial tubercle

A

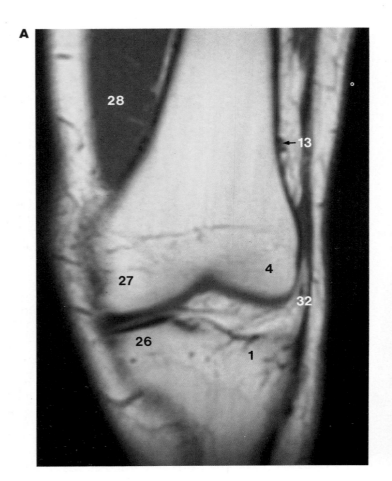

B

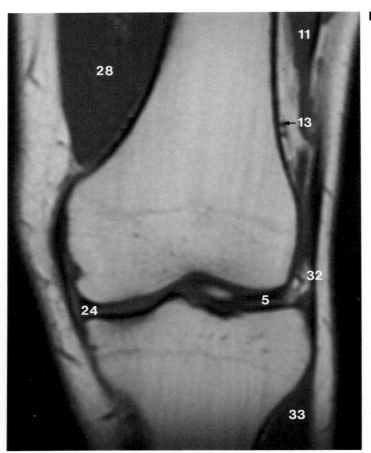

C

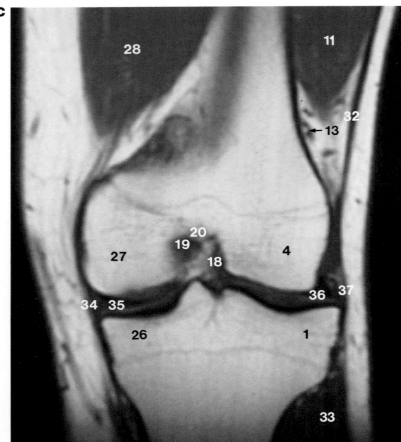

A—F Knee. Coronal MR images (T$_1$-weighted)

1	Lateral condyle of tibia
2	Head of fibula
3	Tibiofibular joint
4	Lateral condyle of femur
5	Anterior ⎫
6	Posterior ⎬ horn of lateral meniscus
7	Patella
8	Tendon of quadriceps muscle
9	Patellar tendon
10	Infrapatellar fat pad
11	Vastus lateralis muscle
12	Short head of biceps femoris muscle
13	Superior lateral genicular artery
14	Lateral head of gastrocnemius muscle
15	Plantaris muscle
16	Popliteus muscle
17	Long head of biceps femoris muscle
18	Anterior cruciate ligament
19	Posterior cruciate ligament
20	Intercondylar notch
21	Popliteal artery and vein
22	Medial head of gastrocnemius muscle
23	Semimembranosus muscle
24	Anterior ⎫
25	Posterior ⎬ horn of medial meniscus

D

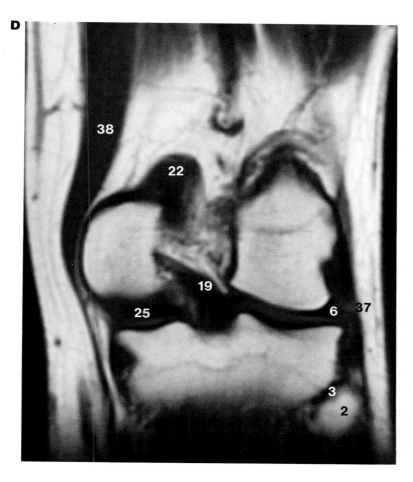

E

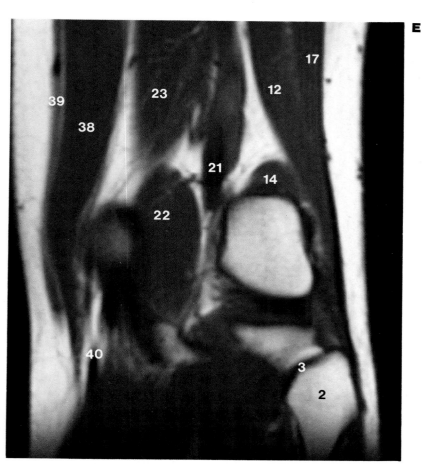

26	Medial condyle of tibia
27	Medial condyle of femur
28	Vastus medialis muscle
29	Posterior meniscofemoral ligament
30	Femur
31	Tibia
32	Iliotibial tract
33	Tibialis anterior muscle
34	Medial collateral ligament
35	Medial ⎫
36	Lateral ⎬ meniscus
37	Lateral collateral ligament
38	Sartorius muscle
39	Gracilis muscle
40	Tendon of semitendinosus muscle
41	Soleus muscle
42	Biceps femoris muscle
43	Common peroneal nerve
44	Great saphenous vein
45	Popliteal artery
46	Popliteal vein
47	Lateral ⎫
48	Medial ⎬ patellar retinaculum
49	Tibial tubercle

F

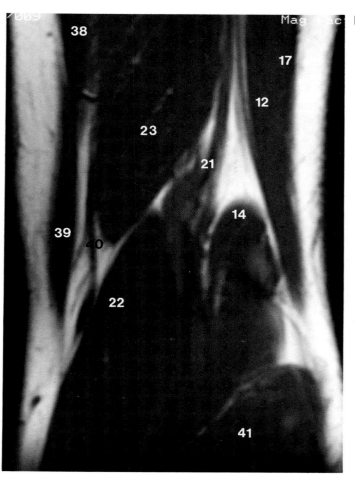

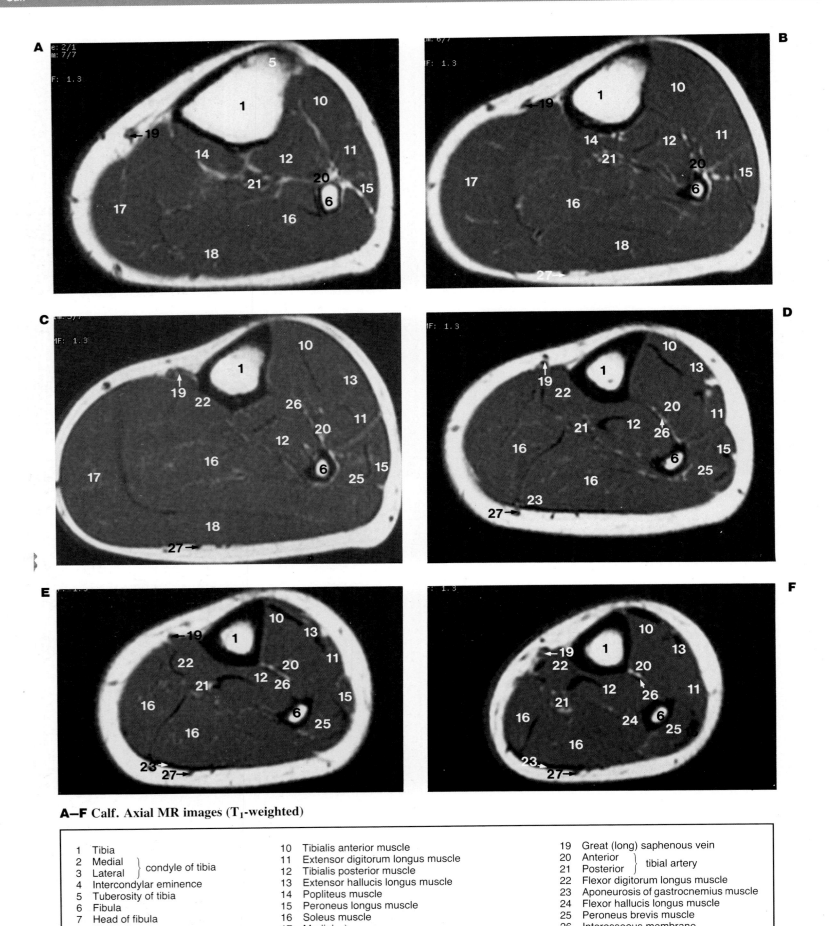

A–F Calf. Axial MR images (T₁-weighted)

1	Tibia	10	Tibialis anterior muscle	19	Great (long) saphenous vein
2	Medial ⎫	11	Extensor digitorum longus muscle	20	Anterior ⎫
3	Lateral ⎬ condyle of tibia	12	Tibialis posterior muscle	21	Posterior ⎬ tibial artery
4	Intercondylar eminence	13	Extensor hallucis longus muscle	22	Flexor digitorum longus muscle
5	Tuberosity of tibia	14	Popliteus muscle	23	Aponeurosis of gastrocnemius muscle
6	Fibula	15	Peroneus longus muscle	24	Flexor hallucis longus muscle
7	Head of fibula	16	Soleus muscle	25	Peroneus brevis muscle
8	Iliotibial tract	17	Medial ⎫	26	Interosseous membrane
9	Patellar tendon	18	Lateral ⎬ head of gastrocnemius muscle	27	Small saphenous vein

A—F Ankle. Axial MR images (T₁-weighted)

1 Tendon of tibialis anterior muscle
2 Extensor hallucis longus muscle
3 Tendon of extensor hallucis longus muscle
4 Extensor digitorum muscle
5 Tendon of extensor digitorum muscle
6 Tibialis posterior muscle
7 Tendon of tibialis posterior muscle
8 Flexor digitorum longus muscle
9 Tendon of flexor digitorum longus muscle
10 Flexor hallucis longus muscle
11 Tendon of flexor hallucis longus muscle
12 Tendon of peroneus longus muscle
13 Peroneus brevis muscle
14 Tendo calcaneus (Achilles' tendon)
15 Tibia
16 Fibula
17 Small saphenous vein
18 Posterior tibial artery and vein
19 Interosseous membrane
20 Great (long) saphenous vein
21 Anterior tibial artery and vein
22 Soleus muscle
23 Peroneus tertius muscle
24 Fibular notch
25 Lateral ⎫
26 Medial ⎬ malleolus
27 Superior surface of talus
28 Inferior tibiofibular joint
29 Deltoid ligament
30 Talus
31 Calcaneus
32 Calcaneal tuberosity
33 Sustentaculum tali
34 Posterior subtalar joint
35 Medial subtalar joint
36 Tarsal sinus
37 Tendon of peroneus brevis muscle
38 Abductor hallucis muscle
39 Neck ⎫
40 Head ⎬ of talus
41 Tendon of peroneus tertius muscle
42 Tendon of extensor digitorum brevis muscle
43 Flexor accessorius muscle
44 Plantar artery and vein
45 Tuberosity of navicular
46 Medial cuneiform
47 First metatarsal
48 Flexor digitorum brevis muscle
49 Navicular
50 Plantar aponeurosis
51 Interosseous talocalcaneal ligament
52 Tibiotalar part of ankle joint
53 Abductor digiti minimi muscle
54 Talonavicular joint
55 Intermediate cuneiform
56 Second metatarsal
57 Cuboid
58 Lateral cuneiform
59 Anterior tubercle of calcaneus
60 Calcaneocuboid joint
61 Cuneonavicular joint
62 Third metatarsal

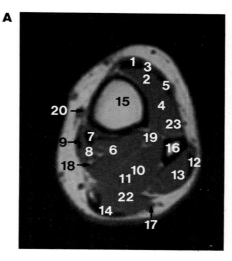
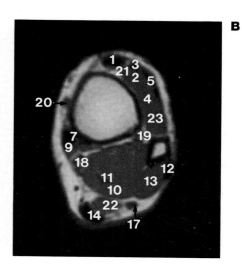
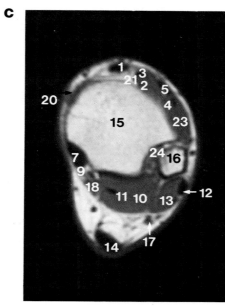
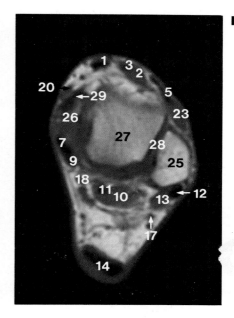
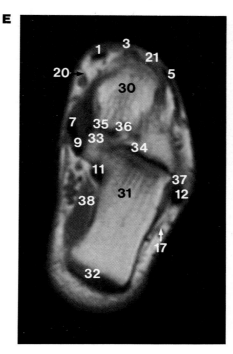
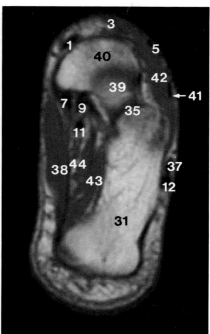

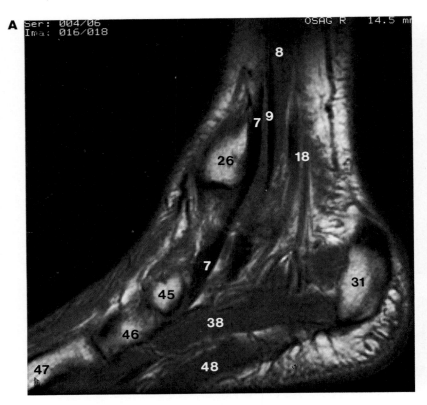

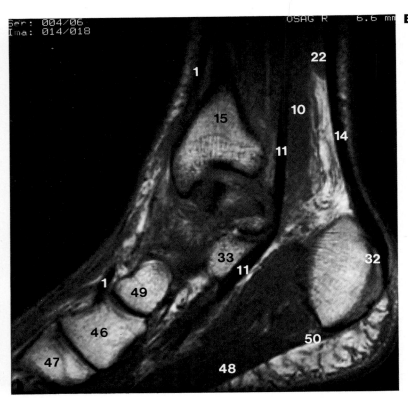

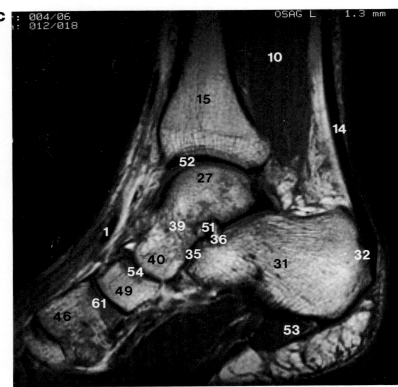

A–F Ankle. Sagittal MR images (T₁-weighted)

$$A-F \text{ Ankle. Sagittal MR images } (T_1\text{-weighted})$$

1. Tendon of tibialis anterior muscle
2. Extensor hallucis longus muscle
3. Tendon of extensor hallucis longus muscle
4. Extensor digitorum muscle
5. Tendon of extensor digitorum muscle
6. Tibialis posterior muscle
7. Tendon of tibialis posterior muscle
8. Flexor digitorum longus muscle
9. Tendon of flexor digitorum longus muscle
10. Flexor hallucis longus muscle
11. Tendon of flexor hallucis longus muscle
12. Tendon of peroneus longus muscle
13. Peroneus brevis muscle
14. Tendo calcaneus (Achilles' tendon)
15. Tibia
16. Fibula
17. Small saphenous vein
18. Posterior tibial artery and vein
19. Interosseous membrane
20. Great (long) saphenous vein
21. Anterior tibial artery and vein
22. Soleus muscle
23. Peroneus tertius muscle
24. Fibular notch
25. Lateral ⎫
26. Medial ⎬ malleolus
27. Superior surface of talus
28. Inferior tibiofibular joint
29. Deltoid ligament
30. Talus
31. Calcaneus

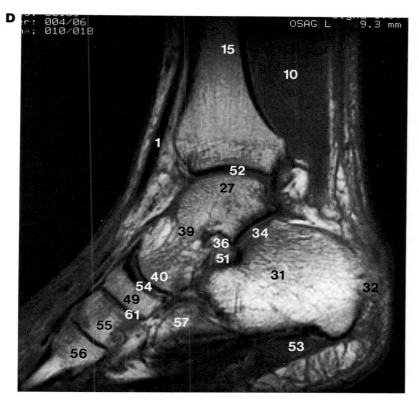

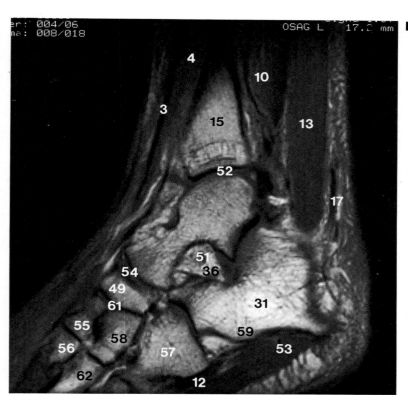

32	Calcaneal tuberosity
33	Sustentaculum tali
34	Posterior subtalar joint
35	Medial subtalar joint
36	Tarsal sinus
37	Tendon of peroneus brevis muscle
38	Abductor hallucis muscle
39	Neck } of talus
40	Head } of talus
41	Tendon of peroneus tertius muscle
42	Tendon of extensor digitorum brevis muscle
43	Flexor accessorius muscle
44	Plantar artery and vein
45	Tuberosity of navicular
46	Medial cuneiform
47	First metatarsal
48	Flexor digitorum brevis muscle
49	Navicular
50	Plantar aponeurosis
51	Interosseous talocalcaneal ligament
52	Tibiotalar part of ankle joint
53	Abductor digiti minimi muscle
54	Talonavicular joint
55	Intermediate cuneiform
56	Second metatarsal
57	Cuboid
58	Lateral cuneiform
59	Anterior tubercle of calcaneus
60	Calcaneocuboid joint
61	Cuneonavicular joint
62	Third metatarsal

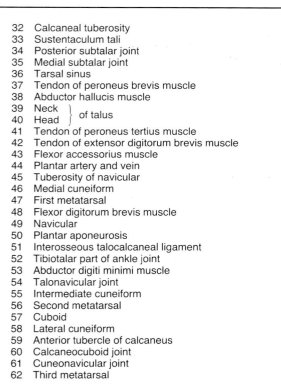

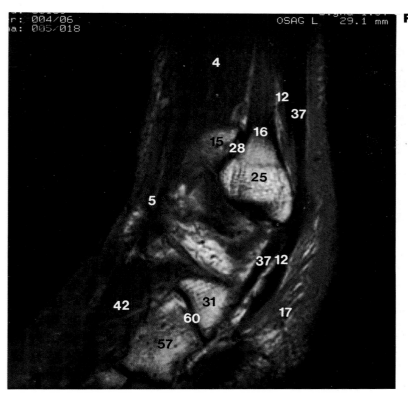

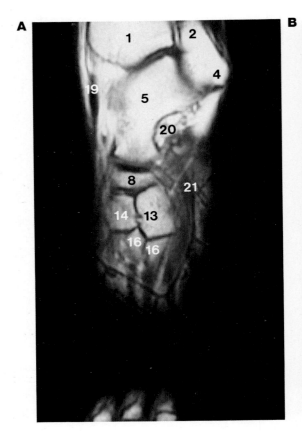

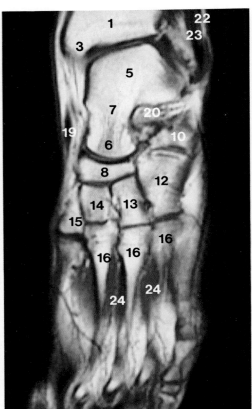

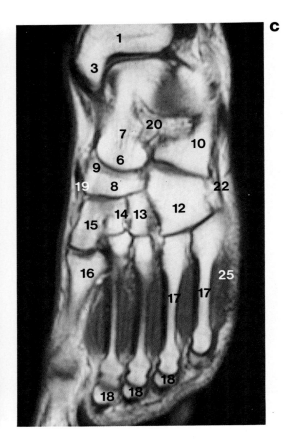

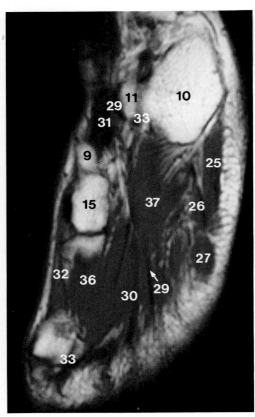

Foot. A—E Oblique axial MR images (T$_1$-weighted), **F—K** coronal MR images (T$_1$-weighted)

1	Tibia
2	Fibula
3	Medial ⎫
4	Lateral ⎬ malleolus
5	Talus
6	Head ⎫
7	Neck ⎬ of talus
8	Navicular
9	Tuberosity of talus
10	Calcaneus
11	Sustentaculum tali
12	Cuboid
13	Lateral ⎫
14	Intermediate ⎬ cuneiform
15	Medial ⎭
16	Base ⎫
17	Shaft ⎬ of metatarsal
18	Base of proximal phalanx
19	Tendon of tibialis anterior muscle
20	Tarsal sinus
21	Extensor digitorum brevis muscle
22	Tendon of peroneus brevis muscle
23	Tendon of peroneus longus muscle
24	Dorsal interossei muscle
25	Abductor digiti minimi muscle
26	Flexor digiti minimi muscle
27	Opponens digiti minimi muscle
28	Adductor hallucis muscle
29	Tendon of flexor digitorum longus muscle

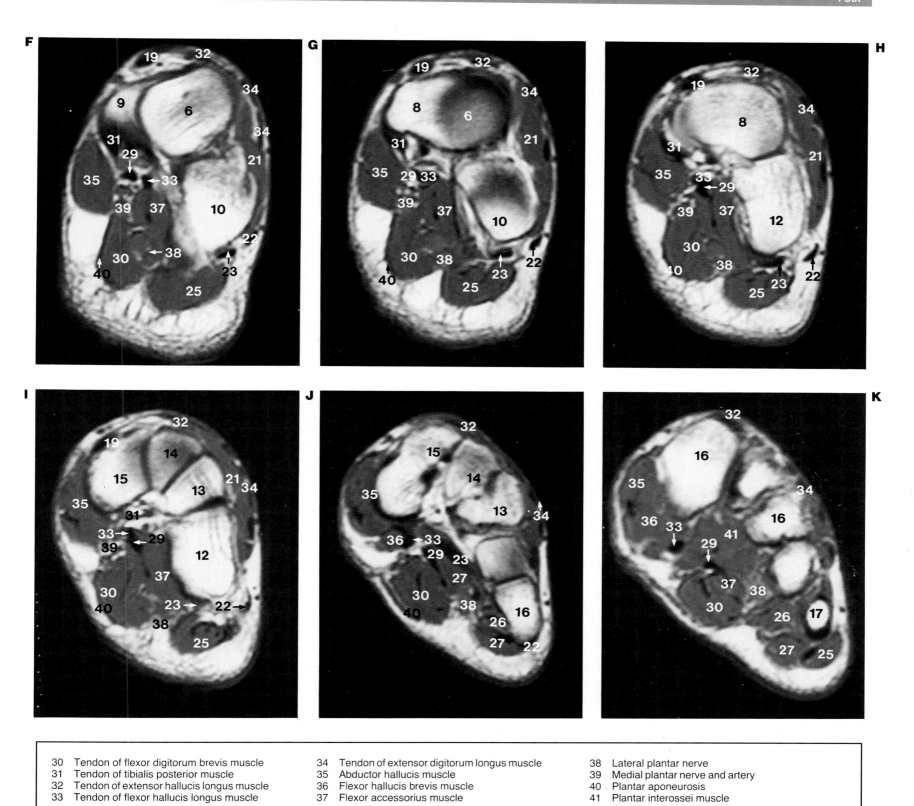

30	Tendon of flexor digitorum brevis muscle	34 Tendon of extensor digitorum longus muscle
31	Tendon of tibialis posterior muscle	35 Abductor hallucis muscle
32	Tendon of extensor hallucis longus muscle	36 Flexor hallucis brevis muscle
33	Tendon of flexor hallucis longus muscle	37 Flexor accessorius muscle

38	Lateral plantar nerve
39	Medial plantar nerve and artery
40	Plantar aponeurosis
41	Plantar interossei muscle

191

INDEX